MW01287261

Pilates for Rehabilitation

Pilates for Rehabilitation

Samantha Wood

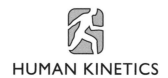

HUMAN KINETICS

Library of Congress Cataloging-in-Publication Data

Names: Wood, Samantha, 1969- author.
Title: Pilates for rehabilitation / Samantha Wood.
Description: Champaign, IL : Human Kinetics, [2019] | Includes
 bibliographical references and index.
Identifiers: LCCN 2018005342 (print) | LCCN 2017058453 (ebook) | ISBN
 9781492556503 (ebook) | ISBN 9781492556497 (print)
Subjects: LCSH: Pilates method. | Physical therapy. | Sports medicine.
Classification: LCC RA781.4 (print) | LCC RA781.4 .W66 2019 (ebook) | DDC
 613.7/192--dc23
LC record available at https://lccn.loc.gov/2018005342

ISBN: 978-1-4925-5649-7 (print)

Copyright © 2019 by Samantha Wood

All rights reserved. Except for use in a review, the reproduction or utilization of this work in any form or by any electronic, mechanical, or other means, now known or hereafter invented, including xerography, photocopying, and recording, and in any information storage and retrieval system, is forbidden without the written permission of the publisher.

This publication is written and published to provide accurate and authoritative information relevant to the subject matter presented. It is published and sold with the understanding that the author and publisher are not engaged in rendering legal, medical, or other professional services by reason of their authorship or publication of this work. If medical or other expert assistance is required, the services of a competent professional person should be sought.

The web addresses cited in this text were current as of April 2018, unless otherwise noted.

Senior Acquisitions Editor: Michelle Maloney; **Managing Editor:** Ann C. Gindes; **Copyeditor:** Janet Kiefer; **Indexer:** Michael Ferreira; **Permissions Manager:** Martha Gullo; **Graphic Designer:** Whitney Milburn; **Cover Designer:** Keri Evans; **Cover Design Associate:** Susan Rothermel Allen; **Photograph (cover):** © Human Kinetics; **Photographs (interior):** © Human Kinetics unless otherwise noted; **Photographer (cover and interior):** Kirk Fitzik; **Cover Models:** Jeff Rozic and Samantha Wood; **Interior photo models:** Alonzo Cannon, Ena Kirima, Sheri Long, Jeff Rozic, and Samantha Wood; **Photo Production Coordinator:** Amy M. Rose; **Photo Production Manager:** Jason Allen; **Senior Art Manager:** Kelly Hendren; **Illustrations:** © Human Kinetics unless otherwise noted; **Printer:** Sheridan Books

We thank BASI Pilates International Headquarters in Costa Mesa, California, for assistance in providing the location for the photo shoot for this book.

Human Kinetics books are available at special discounts for bulk purchase. Special editions or book excerpts can also be created to specification. For details, contact the Special Sales Manager at Human Kinetics.

Printed in the United States of America   10   9   8   7   6   5   4   3   2

The paper in this book is certified under a sustainable forestry program.

Human Kinetics
P.O. Box 5076
Champaign, IL 61825-5076
Website: www.HumanKinetics.com

In the United States, email info@hkusa.com or call 800-747-4457.
In Canada, email info@hkcanada.com.
In the United Kingdom/Europe, email hk@hkeurope.com.

For information about Human Kinetics' coverage in other areas of the world,
please visit our website: **www.HumanKinetics.com**

E7110

Tell us what you think!
Human Kinetics would love to hear what we
can do to improve the customer experience.
Use this QR code to take our brief survey.

DEDICATION

I dedicate this book to my mom, Joni Gray. She always believed that you can do anything if you just put your mind to it. She was a living example of courage, strength, and love. Always my biggest fan, she was so excited to tell everyone that her daughter was writing a book! It breaks my heart that she is not here to see the finished product. I hope she is looking down with pride.

I would also like to dedicate this book to Rael Isacowitz—my teacher, my mentor, and, most importantly, my friend. Without his teachings, encouragement, and ongoing support, this book would have never happened. Rael's dedication to the Pilates method and his generous sharing of his knowledge and experience through his courses and books is a true inspiration. For his graciousness in allowing me to include his original exercises and eloquent words in my practice and in this book, I am forever grateful. It has been an honor to study under him and to work alongside him. I look forward to continuing our journey.

CONTENTS

PART I   THE CASE FOR PILATES

1 The Science Behind Pilates for Rehabilitation   2

Discover recent studies that show how Pilates can be an effective tool for injury rehabilitation.

2 Guiding Principles of Pilates   14

Explore the foundation of Pilates as a unique form of conditioning for the mind and the body.

3 Integrating Pilates With Rehabilitation   22

Guide patients from earlier stages of physiotherapy to long-term conditioning by optimizing alignment and creating correct movement patters with Pilates.

4 Methodology and Apparatus Needed for an Effective Practice   36

Understand how the combination of Pilates methods, therapeutic concepts, and usage of a variety of equipment options leads to maximum movement potential.

PART II EXERCISES

FOREWORD

I began delving into Pilates in the late 1970s. I cannot say that I immediately became a devotee of the system; that did not happen for several years. However, I immediately saw tremendous value in the Pilates method. Since an early age I had been involved in athletic and movement pursuits. These included swimming competitively, practicing yoga, and studying dance. I have always had a deep love of nature and the outdoors, so surfing, windsurfing, mountain biking, skiing, snowboarding, and, most recently, kiteboarding and standup paddling are all dear to my heart. My bachelor's degree was in physical education (Wingate Institute, Israel) with a strong emphasis on exercise physiology and biomechanics. I subsequently joined the faculty at Wingate for several years. I had a strong fascination with the science of human movement, and this was the thrust of my studies. Yet I became increasingly drawn to dance and the art of movement. This led to a long career as a dancer and to completing my master's degree in dance studies (University of Surrey, England). By the mid-1980s I started recognizing the immense and unique value that Pilates could have for extremely diverse populations. It was this diversity that captured my imagination, and probably that of many others, as witnessed by the astronomical growth of Pilates in the early part of the new millennium.

I moved from England to Australia in 1989; after working almost exclusively with dancers, I also started working very closely with top level athletes of other disciplines. Inevitably, my path merged with physical therapists, physicians, osteopaths, chiropractors, and others who were treating the dancers and athletes. Pilates became the meeting ground, the common denominator, the comprehensive exercise program that all these professions ultimately longed for. It was particularly with the physical therapists that I formed a very close working relationship and bond.

Upon arriving in the United States in 1991 at the invitation of an orthopedic surgeon, I strived to continue this exciting multifaceted approach to well-being. However, I was witnessing an interesting and somewhat disturbing trend. Physical therapists were adopting Pilates and integrating it into their practices. (With its growing popularity, they could hardly afford not to.) Yet they were not embracing the system itself. They were taking select pieces of apparatus, choosing some isolated exercises from the vast repertoire, and claiming to teach Pilates. Some were even declaring that you needed to be a qualified physical therapist to study and practice this "unique" type of Pilates. Joseph Pilates, the inventor of this method, was *not* a physical therapist. Nor were the very talented first-generation teachers I'd had the distinct pleasure and honor of studying with.

I longed to collaborate with a highly skilled and educated physical therapist to create a two-way bridge between Pilates practitioners and physical therapists. As the popularity of Pilates continued to grow, Pilates practitioners needed more knowledge of injuries and pathologies. They needed guidance, and still do, as to how to use the hundreds of exercises and build effective programs for specific needs. On the other hand, physical therapists needed to study this vast system and not just select pieces of the system. This process of splintering Pilates was resulting in its losing what made it so attractive to physical therapists and medical practitioners in the first place—its comprehensive nature.

I was fortunate to be introduced to Samantha (Sam) Wood by my wife in the mid-1990s. The fact that Sam was highly intelligent, skilled, and extremely well educated did not take me long to uncover. Yet what impressed me most from the very outset was Sam's drive to study Pilates from the ground up; she did not assume that she already knew Pilates by virtue of the fact that she was a physical therapist. The fact that Sam had spent years broadening her movement experience by studying yoga gave us common ground, and she could relate to what had become the BASI (Body Arts and Science International) approach: a holistic view of Pilates, integrating body, mind, and spirit—as Mr. Joseph H. Pilates had intended. The power of the body is finite, but the power that lies within the mind knows no bounds.

Sam and I discussed at length my vision, which soon became our shared vision. She did not hesitate to dive in and complete the BASI comprehensive training, a rigorous and demanding program. She then went on to complete the Legacy Program of BASI teacher training. Sam devoted years to honing her Pilates skills, just as she had done with her physical therapy skills. She then went on to integrate the two in the most perfect union of the two disciplines that I have witnessed to date. The results speak for themselves.

As part of our vision, Sam created (with my guidance and input) an advanced course of study titled Injuries and Pathologies. Sam has taught this course worldwide with an overwhelming response and resounding acclaim. The exercises presented in this course are adapted from the vast body of work taught in our programs, which include both the classic Pilates exercises and many of my own creations. Sam masterfully adapted the repertoire, even the highest-level repertoire, to the needs of the select populations she was addressing.

So when Human Kinetics, the publisher of two of my books, *Pilates* and *Pilates Anatomy* (coauthored with Karen Clippinger), approached me for recommendations of a potential author for a Pilates book geared toward working with injuries and pathologies, it did not take long for me to recommend my friend and colleague Samantha Wood.

BASI is a contemporary, evidence-based approach to a phenomenal system that was gifted to us by Joseph and Clara Pilates—a method of physical and mental conditioning that has touched and changed so many lives. When asked how it works, we are tempted to just say, "It works. We don't know why, and we don't need to know how; just do it, and you will see the results!" However, the fact is that we *do* need to strive to understand. We need to glean information from research and from therapists working on the cutting edge. We need to bring together the hundreds of cumulative years of experience of practitioners with the academic knowledge of young, brilliant minds graduating from universities around the globe.

Pilates is a comprehensive method with the ultimate goal of achieving well-being. Interestingly Joseph Pilates seldom, if ever, spoke of *just* exercise. The exercises are vehicles toward the ultimate goal of physical, mental, and spiritual health and harmony. To ignore this holistic view is to ignore the very foundation and tenets of Pilates. Samantha has created a book that honors this view while integrating her many years of experience in the field of physical therapy and her vast knowledge of human science. Whether you are a physical therapist, Pilates practitioner, Pilates enthusiast, or athlete, or you are simply interested in learning about integrating Pilates successfully into the world of therapy, you will undoubtedly benefit from this important and profound book.

—Rael Isacowitz

ACKNOWLEDGMENTS

I would like to thank everyone on the Human Kinetics team who helped with this book. A special thanks to Michelle Maloney, my acquisitions editor, for her patient guidance, enthusiastic encouragement, and valuable critiques. A kinder person I cannot imagine. And I thank Ann Gindes, my managing editor, for her belief in this book and help improving it through the editing process.

A huge thank you to my wonderful and talented models, Alonzo Cannon, Ena Kirima, Sheri Long, and Jeff Rozic. Their skills, time, and enthusiasm for being a part of this book are so appreciated.

I would like to express my appreciation to Kirk Fitzik for his excellent photography. His extensive experience in working with Pilates teachers was so valuable. The photo shoot flowed smoothly thanks to his professionalism, artful eye, and helpful suggestions.

I wish to acknowledge BASI Pilates International Headquarters for allowing us to use their beautiful studio and the amazing BASI Systems Pilates equipment. The assistance provided by Stella Hull-Lampkin in coordinating the logistics was greatly appreciated.

I would also like to thank the many people who have helped validate and fine-tune the exercises in this book: the patients who have been willing to let me rehabilitate their injuries with Pilates, and the Pilates teachers and rehabilitation professionals who have participated in my courses and workshops over the years. It has been a privilege to work with and learn from all of them—they are the inspiration for this book!

Special thanks to my business partner and friend, Rachel Clark, for making it easy for me to take time away from our wellness center to work on this project. I am so grateful for her patience, kindness, support, and encouragement. And I appreciate her willingness to share her knowledge and the valuable suggestions for improvement she provided.

Finally, a big thanks to my support team at home who kept me sane throughout this process: Jeff and Kai. I am so grateful for their patience and love each and every day.

INTRODUCTION

As a physical therapist who specializes in Pilates-based rehabilitation, I don't typically work with patients whose goal is getting fit. My patients come because of a specific injury or pathology that is limiting their activities. At my wellness center in Pacific Palisades, California, we have been integrating Pilates into patient treatments for over 16 years, with excellent outcomes. I have witnessed firsthand that Pilates can be a highly effective tool for therapeutic purposes when used appropriately, and research supports those findings. Pilates exercises and principles can help patients recover from injuries and surgery as well as optimize function in patients suffering from chronic conditions. The Pilates method helps manage the pain and dysfunction experienced by many patients, especially when it is combined with traditional physical therapy or other rehabilitation techniques.

Why is this? Pilates is not just a physical process; it's a mind–body form of conditioning. I have seen many patients over the years reach far greater potential when mental conditioning is integrated into the motor learning and neuromuscular reeducation process. Pilates is not simply exercise; it is a holistic approach to optimizing human movement (Isacowitz 2014). Pilates is versatile and adaptable, so it is appropriate for nearly any patient or client. It offers a solution to individuals across the spectrum of mobility and fitness—from the 93-year-old woman with osteoporosis and a total hip arthroplasty to the professional athlete with an ACL reconstruction. It is as motivating for men as for women, and it is safe for all ages when used correctly.

What is Pilates? It is a method of exercise based on the work of a man named Joseph Pilates. His guiding philosophy in creating the apparatus and the movements was that the whole must be exercised to achieve good health. There is a large repertoire of movements on each piece of apparatus, developing from fundamental level to master level. Using springs and pulleys, which create progressive resistance, the equipment helps produce both concentric and eccentric muscle contractions that simulate functional muscle action. At the same time, the stabilizing muscle groups are encouraged to work isometrically to maintain correct positioning and alignment.

Glenn Withers, founder of the Australian Physiotherapy and Pilates Institute, recounts that Joseph Pilates believed that injuries were caused by imbalances in the body and habitual patterns of movement; when a person had a weakness or malaligned area, an overcompensation or overdevelopment of another area occurred in order to achieve the functional movement desired. Joseph felt it was critical to correct the malalignment and to reeducate the body in order to prevent recurrence. Over 50 years later, this theory of muscle imbalance is widely accepted in the field of physiotherapy (Withers and Bryant 2011).

Joseph Pilates was clearly a man ahead of his time. Born in Dusseldorf, Germany, in 1883, he had rickets, asthma, and rheumatic fever as a child. Attempting to overcome these ailments, he took up various types of physical fitness:

bodybuilding, gymnastics, diving, martial arts, and yoga. During World War I he was interned in a POW camp on the Isle of Man. While there, he taught and practiced his physical fitness program. It was in this camp that he began devising apparatus to aid in the rehabilitation of the disabled and sick.

After the war, Joseph left for America by boat. On the voyage, he met Clara, who later became his wife. In 1926, Joseph and Clara Pilates set up the first Pilates studio in New York City. Over the course of his career, Joseph Pilates developed over 600 exercises for the various pieces of apparatus he invented. He designed the equipment to condition the entire body using positions and movements that would correct body alignment and balance. Joseph wanted his method (which he called *contrology*) taught in every school, and he felt that the medical profession should embrace the physical and mental benefits of his work (Isacowitz 2014). Unfortunately, he died in 1967 before his method became well known and widely accepted.

Decades later, numerous articles have been published in medical journals advocating the use of Pilates in rehabilitation. The two primary benefits often mentioned are improved neuromuscular control of the intrinsic core and performance enhancement. As physical therapists, we are always searching for a system that can take patients from the early stages of rehabilitation to the long-term goal of a conditioned, efficiently functioning body. Pilates is that system! Other rehabilitation professionals often ask me why I am such a believer in the Pilates method. Chapter 3 goes into more detail on this, but the following is a summary of the method's selling points:

- Pilates focuses on the core muscles (also called the *powerhouse*).
- Pilates exercises emphasize both stability and mobility.
- Pilates includes both closed kinetic chain and open kinetic chain exercises.
- Pilates exercises work muscles statically and dynamically, emphasizing both concentric and eccentric muscular contractions.
- Pilates exercises are functional.
- Pilates places an importance on breathing appropriately.
- Pilates is a mind–body form of conditioning.
- Pilates is adaptable for many different patient populations.
- Pilates equipment is safe and easy to use (with proper training).
- Pilates is a wise business choice for anyone wishing to expand their wellness services.

If you are not yet well versed in the method but have seen some of the more classical Pilates exercises performed, you might doubt that these could be appropriate for injury rehabilitation. Indeed, many of the exercises must be modified for rehabilitative purposes—in some cases severely. My approach with patients is as follows: Exercises are chosen and sequenced based on the specific needs of the patient, while attempting to maintain the holistic approach of the work. Exercises are not changed to accommodate movements the person may be accustomed to; instead, the individual adapts to corrections and positive movement patterns being taught. The goal then becomes achieving optimal posture, functional strength, and balance in the individual as well as rehabilitating the injury.

The purpose of this book is to familiarize orthopedic rehabilitation professionals with the Pilates philosophy and teach them how to use Pilates as therapeutic exercise with specific patient populations. Whether it's used with fitness enthusiasts, elite athletes, weekend warriors, desk jockeys, or geriatrics, Pilates can benefit all patients and clients. Yes, it can be used to rehabilitate and heal injuries, but it also can increase overall fitness level, improve performance, and provide safe and effective cross-training in the off-season.

The methodology and philosophical approach in this book, as well as the majority of the exercises presented, are gleaned from the work of Rael Isacowitz and the Body Arts and Science International (BASI) Pilates courses. I took my first Pilates training course with Rael in 1999; since then I have completed all of BASI's programs, including Rael's Legacy Program, which includes the Mentor, Master I, and Master II courses. Some of the exercises chosen for this book are based on classical Pilates, but a many are Rael's exercises, which I have then modified to be suitable for the purpose of injury rehabilitation.

In part I, the rationale behind Pilates for rehabilitation and how it differs from a traditional Pilates practice are explained. This part reviews the guiding principles, examines the tenets of Pilates, and establishes why and how Pilates can be an invaluable tool for rehab professionals to have in their toolboxes.

Part II presents the physical movements of the Pilates exercises. There are over 600 exercises in classical Pilates alone, so I have only selected those exercises I feel are most beneficial for rehabilitation of common orthopedic injuries. Accordingly, pathological indications and contraindications, muscle focus, and biomechanical and neuromuscular considerations are addressed in relation to each exercise. Movements are described with detailed instructions, and modifications and progressions are presented as appropriate.

Part III puts it all together. Exercise programs that can be used for specific injuries and pathologies are offered. The content is organized by anatomical region: cervical spine and thoracic spine, lumbar spine, shoulder, hip, knee, and foot and ankle.

Pilates for Rehabilitation provides a Pilates resource for physical therapists, physical therapy assistants, chiropractors, athletic trainers, personal trainers, and Pilates teachers. Although I highly recommend investing in a comprehensive Pilates education from a reputable school, by the time you are finished with this book you will have the tools to begin to integrate Pilates effectively into treatment plans for all your patients and clients.

THE CASE
FOR PILATES

1

The Science Behind Pilates for Rehabilitation

Over the last decade and a half, there has been a growing body of literature published in medical journals advocating the use of the Pilates method as an effective form of conservative treatment for injury rehabilitation in the field of physiotherapy. Pilates has been shown to improve core strength (Emery et al. 2010; Kloubec 2010), increase muscle strength and overall flexibility (Kao et al. 2015; Kloubec 2010; Campos de Oliveira, Goncalves de Oliveria and Pires-Oliveria 2015; Sekendiz et al. 2007; Segal, Hein, and Basford 2004), promote efficient movement (Emery et al. 2010; Herrington and Davies 2005), improve posture and enhance postural balance (Alves de Araujo et al. 2012; Emery et al. 2010; Natour et al. 2015; Campos de Oliveira, Goncalves de Oliveria and Pires-Oliveria 2015), restore function, and help to manage pain (Campos de Oliveira, Goncalves de Oliveria and Pires-Oliveria 2015; Rydeard et al. 2006; Wells et al. 2014). For the benefit of those who need to see scientific evidence, the following pages summarize some of the best work published thus far.

Pilates for the Core

Because all movement originates from the *center* or *core* (more on this later), this seems a logical place to begin. The importance of the deepest abdominal muscle, the transversus abdominis (TrA), as a spinal stabilizer has been well established, both in the literature and in clinical practice. In patients with low back pain, we often see delayed onset of muscle activity of the TrA with movement of the limbs in all directions, and this change in TrA control occurs irrespective of the specific pathology (Hodges and Richardson 1996, 1998). Thus, retraining the TrA to increase spinal stabilization is a widely accepted concept in lumbo-pelvic pain rehabilitation (Comerford and Mottram 2001; Hodges and Richardson 1999). In addition to the TrA, the other deep muscles that attach directly to the trunk and offer stabilization (often referred to as the "local muscle system") are the lumbar multifidi, the diaphragm, and the pelvic floor muscles.

In recent years, there has been increased focus on the management of chronic low back pain from a motor control perspective, rather than from a pure strength perspective. In 2000, Jull and Richardson published a study in the *Journal of Manipulative Physiological Therapy* in which they called for a new direction for therapeutic exercises—one that is based on research into muscle dysfunction in patients with low back pain that has led to discoveries of impairments in the deep muscles of the trunk and back. They pointed out that these muscles have a functional role in enhancing spinal segmental support and control of the spine and that the muscle impairments seen in patients with spinal pain are in motor control, not strength. Their specific exercise approach has an initial focus on retraining the cocontraction of the deep muscles attached to the spine. Their results showed that this approach is effective in reducing neuromuscular impairment and in controlling pain in patients with both acute and chronic low back pain.

How do we activate these deep muscles of the trunk? The abdominal drawing-in maneuver (ADIM) is a fundamental exercise in traditional stabilization programs for lower back pain. The ADIM is often used to facilitate the reeducation of neuromuscular control mechanisms provided by the deep local stabilizing muscles (Richardson, Jull, and Hodges 2004; Urquhart et al 2005). It has been established that during an abdominal draw-in pattern, the multifidus muscle cocontracts with the TrA muscle (Richardson et al. 2002). A 2011 study by Hides and colleagues showed that having a poor TrA contraction was related to a poor ability to contract the multifidus, whereas patients who had a strong contraction of the TrA were four and a half times more likely to have a strong contraction of the multifidus. Additionally, electromyogram studies by Sapsford and colleagues (2001) have shown that abdominal muscle activity is a normal response to pelvic floor exercise in subjects without pelvic floor muscle dysfunction and that submaximal isometric abdominal exercises activate the pelvic floor muscles. Therefore the key to recruiting all of these muscles seems to be the TrA.

So what does all of this have to do with Pilates? Pilates exercises involve activation of the deep, local stabilizing muscles of the trunk via an imprint action. Though perhaps cued differently, this action is basically the same as the ADIM proven to activate the TrA in spinal stabilization training. It follows, then, that Pilates exercises would be effective in stabilizing the lumbar spine and thus in treating lumbo-pelvic pain via improving the neuromuscular control of these deep muscles with this drawing-in or imprint action. But is there evidence to support this claim? Does the imprint action in Pilates exercises activate the deep abdominal muscles? Yes, it does, as evidenced by the studies explained here.

Pilates Research Review: The Core

Pilates and Activation of the Deep Abdominals

A 2008 study by Endleman and Critchley provided the first evidence that specific Pilates exercises activate the deeper abdominal muscles. The researchers used ultrasound imaging to measure the thickness change of the transversus abdominis (TrA) and obliquus internus (OI) when subjects performed a representative set of classical Pilates exercises: imprint, hundred, roll-up, leg circle on the mat, and hundred on the reformer. The researchers found a significant increase in thickness, representing muscle activity, in both TrA and OI during all correctly performed Pilates exercises compared with resting supine. Another interesting finding was that TrA thickness during the hundred exercise (p. 67) was greater than when performed on a mat, demonstrating that use of the reformer can result in greater TrA activation in some exercises.

Endleman, I. and D. J. Critchley. 2008. Transversus abdominis and obliquus internus activity during Pilates exercises: Measurement with ultrasound scanning. *Archives of Physical Medicine and Rehabilitation* 89: 2205-12.

Pilates and Lumbo-Pelvic Control

A 2005 study by Herrington and Davies provided evidence that Pilates-trained subjects could contract the TrA and maintain better lumbo-pelvic control than those who perform regular abdominal curl exercises or no abdominal muscle exercises. The researchers used a pressure biofeedback unit to assess performance of the TrA muscle during an abdominal hollowing activity (TrA isolation test) and under limb load (lumbo-pelvic stability test) on three groups of asymptomatic females: 12 were Pilates trained, 12 did abdominal curl exercises regularly, and the remaining 12 were the nontraining control group.

Of the 17 subjects who passed the TrA isolation test, 10 were from the Pilates-trained group (83 percent passing rate), 4 were from the abdominal curl group (33 percent), and 3 were from the control group (25 percent). Only 5 of the 36 subjects (14 percent) passed the lumbo-pelvic stability test, and they were all from the Pilates-trained group! All subjects from the abdominal curl and control groups failed the lumbo-pelvic stability test.

Herrington, L., and R. Davies. 2005. The influence of Pilates training on the ability to contract the transversus abdominis muscle in asymptomatic individuals. *Journal of Bodywork and Movement Therapies* 9 (1): 52-57.

Pilates for Nonspecific Chronic Low Back Pain

So far the studies reviewed have shown that Pilates exercises are effective in recruiting the deep spinal stabilizers in asymptomatic individuals. But do Pilates exercises have the same effect on people with low back pain?

Pilates Research Review: Pilates for Chronic Low Back Pain

Pilates for Treating Chronic Low Back Pain

Rydeard, Leger, and Smith conducted a randomized controlled trial in 2006 to investigate the effectiveness of Pilates-based therapeutic exercise on pain and functional disability in a population with nonspecific chronic lower back pain.

In this study, 39 physically active subjects between 20 and 55 years of age were randomly assigned to an exercise-training group and a control group. The exercise-training group did a four-week treatment protocol consisting of specific Pilates exercises on a mat and reformer three days per week in the clinic and a 15-minute home exercise program six days per week. The control group received no specific exercise training and continued with usual care, defined as consultation with a physician and other specialists as necessary. They were instructed to continue with their previous physical activities.

Results showed a significantly lower level of functional disability and average pain intensity in the Pilates group than in the control group following the four-week treatment intervention period. The disability scores in the Pilates group were maintained over the 12-month follow-up period. The main finding of this study was that a program of specific exercise directed at retraining neuromuscular control based on the Pilates method was more efficacious in reducing pain intensity and functional disability levels compared to usual care or no intervention. It is interesting to note, however, that all subjects participating in this study had received treatment for their low back pain in the past. Most of them (90 percent) had tried physiotherapy, 74 percent of which included exercise therapy of some type. So although not specifically investigated or proven in this study, it stands to reason that for this typical active population of people who have nonspecific low back pain, the Pilates-based exercises were more effective than other types of exercise and treatment in decreasing their pain and functional disability.

Rydeard R., A. Leger, and D. Smith. 2006. Pilates-based therapeutic exercise: Effect on subjects with nonspecific chronic low back pain and functional disability: A randomized controlled trial. *Journal of Orthopaedic & Sports Physical Therapy* 36 (7): 472-84.

Pilates and Quality of Life for Chronic Low Back Pain Patients

Another study published in 2015 in *Clinical Rehabilitation* aimed to assess the effectiveness of the Pilates method on pain, function, and quality of life among patients with chronic nonspecific low back pain. The researchers selected 60 patients from a physical therapy waiting list and randomly assigned them to either the experimental group or the control group. Both groups maintained medication treatment with use of nonsteroidal anti-inflammatory drugs (NSAIDs). The experimental group took classes in a Pilates studio twice per week for 90 days.

At four intervals during the study (baseline, 45 days, 90 days, and 180 days) the following parameters were blindly assessed: pain, function, quality of life, satisfaction of treatment, flexibility, and NSAID intake. Comparison between the two groups over time showed a significant difference favoring the Pilates group regarding pain, function, and some quality of life domains. The patients in the Pilates group used less medication and gradually reduced their intake, whereas the control group patients took the same amount of NSAIDs through the end of the study.

From these results, Natour et al. concluded that the Pilates method was effective in reducing pain and improving function and quality of life in patients with chronic, nonspecific low back pain. Further, they pointed out that the Pilates exercises did not worsen pain in the experimental group, demonstrating that use of this method had no harmful effects, and adding support to the belief that Pilates is a safe exercise option for low back pain patients.

Natour, J., L. Araujo Cazotti, L. H. Ribeiro, A. S. Baptista, and A. Jones. 2015. Pilates improves pain, function and quality of life in patients with chronic low back pain: A randomized controlled trial. *Clinical Rehabilitation* 29 (1): 59-68.

Pilates for Specific Low Back Injuries

The studies reviewed thus far have shown that Pilates is effective for chronic, nonspecific low back pain, but is it also effective in a specific, traumatic injury such as spondylolisthesis?

Pilates Research Review: Pilates for Specific Low Back Injuries

Case Study: Traumatic L4–L5 Spondylolisthesis

A 2016 case study by Oliveira, Guedes, Jassi, Martini and Oliveira looked at the effects of the Pilates method on a patient with traumatic L4–L5 spondylolisthesis. This is a rare condition in which one vertebra (most commonly L5–S1) slides anteriorly or posteriorly over another. Surgical intervention is often recommended, but if the patient presents a stable framework (Wells et al. 2014), then conservative techniques that provide improved lumbo-pelvic stability, such as the Pilates method, can be considered.

In the study, three times per week for 12 weeks, the subject, a 45-year-old male, performed a 60-minute sequence of specific Pilates exercises using the ladder barrel, Cadillac, and reformer. The patient was guided by the instructor to follow well-known Pilates principles (see chapter 2). Pre- and posttesting was done to evaluate muscular resistance of the trunk flexor and extensor muscles, strength of the knee flexors and extensors, hip and torso flexibility, postural balance, and pain level.

After 12 weeks, test results demonstrated significant improvement in all variables except for postural balance, which showed only mild improvement. The authors concluded that the Pilates method was effective for improving muscle resistance and strength, flexibility, postural balance, and pain in a patient with traumatic spondylolisthesis at L4–L5. They pointed out that because the Pilates method is a conservative and low-cost treatment, it can be a good option for treatment of patients who present a stable framework of traumatic spondylolisthesis.

Oliveira, L. C., C.A. Guedes, F.J. Jassi, F.A.N. Martini, and R.G. Oliveira. 2016. Effects of the Pilates method on variables related to functionality of a patient with traumatic spondylolisthesis at L4-L5: A case study. *Journal of Bodywork and Movement Therapies* 20 (1): 123-31.

Pilates for the Upper Body

The research presented thus far has focused on the lower spine and the effectiveness of Pilates for injury rehabilitation of lumbo-pelvic dysfunctions. But what about the upper body? Are Pilates exercises also beneficial for those suffering from cervical spine or shoulder pathologies? Though scientific studies on the use of Pilates for what I refer to as the upper core are not as prevalent as for the lower core (lumbo-pelvic region), it is exciting to see more research being published recently. Most researchers credit the positive effects of Pilates seen in patients with upper core injuries to increased cervical stabilization, improved posture, and adherence to Pilates principles such as breathing and focus on coactivation of core muscles (see chapter 2).

Chronic neck pain affects 11 percent to 20 percent of working adults (Cote et al. 2008) and the prevalence and impact of it is increasing (Hoy et al. 2014). Neck pain has been associated with an inefficiency in the cervical stabilizing muscles (deep cervical flexors), which can lead to compensatory increased use and strength of the superficial muscles of the neck and shoulder girdle (Moffett and McClean 2006). Weakness or dysfunction in these upper core, or cervical stabilizing muscles, causes muscle fatigue under sustained low loads, such as sitting in front of a computer or staring down at a smartphone for long periods of time. Cervical stabilization exercises have been shown to improve cervical muscle performance as well as decrease neck pain and headaches (Jull et al. 2002).

In addition to the inhibition and weakness of the deep neck flexors, several studies point to poor thoracic posture, abnormal shoulder biomechanics, and scapular instability as a cause or effect of neck–shoulder disorders (Emery et al. 2010). Stability around the shoulder blades is crucial for efficient movement of the arms and neck. Reeducation of the postural (upper core) muscles of the spine and shoulder girdle may be achieved using specific stabilization exercises, including Pilates (Moffett and McClean 2006).

Pilates Research Review: The Cervical Spine and Shoulder

Pilates for Treating Forward Head Posture

In 2016, the *Journal of Physical Therapy Science* published a study suggesting that Pilates should be recommended as an appropriate method for treatment and prevention of forward head posture (FHP). FHP is becoming more prevalent due to the amount of time people spend looking at electronic devices such as smartphones, tablets, and computers. FHP is clinically defined as the anterior positioning of the cervical spine, and it is associated with neck pain, tension headaches, fatigue, muscle imbalance, and reduced motion of the cervical spine. It is often the precursor to pathologies such as herniated cervical disk, chronic low back pain, and temporomandibular joint dysfunction. Based on previous studies by Kuo, Tully, and Galea (2009), which reported that Pilates can improve thoracic kyphosis in older adults, the authors hypothesized that Pilates may improve cervical spine health by alleviating FHP.

In the study, 28 sedentary female subjects between 23 and 39 years of age with FHP were randomly assigned to either a Pilates group or a combined exercises group. Each group performed exercises 50 minutes per day, three days per week, with added load each week for 10 weeks. The Pilates group exercise program focused on stretching of the neck extensors and pectoral muscles and strengthening of the deep neck flexors, shoulder retractors, back muscles, and abdominal muscles with coactivation of the core muscles by focusing on breathing technique. The combined exercises group's exercise program consisted of stretching and strengthening exercises typically used to improve posture, though without coactivation of the core muscles.

To quantify the amount of FHP in each subject, the craniovertebral angle was measured via cervical spine X-ray. Other pre- and postintervention outcomes measured were cervical range of motion (ROM); muscle fatigue of the upper trapezius, C4 paraspinals, and sternocleidomastoid via surface electromyogram; and subjective reports of pain and disability via the visual analog scale and neck disability index questionnaire.

After the 10 weeks, both groups reported decreased pain and disability levels. However, only the Pilates group showed significant improvement in both craniovertebral angle and cervical ROM. In addition, the Pilates group showed a significant reduction in sternocleidomastoid fatigue, whereas the combined exercise group did not show reduced muscle fatigue in any of the muscles measured, and in fact had increased upper trapezius muscle fatigue.

The authors concluded that the Pilates program was more effective in improving craniovertebral angle (and therefore alleviating FHP), increasing cervical ROM, and decreasing muscle fatigue than the combination of stretching and resistance exercises. They felt that this is due to the focus on strengthening the core muscles in Pilates, which improves overall posture and postural awareness, thereby increasing both global and local stability.

Lee S., C. Lee, D. O'Sullivan, J. Jung, and J. Park. Clinical effectiveness of a Pilates treatment for forward head posture. *Journal of Physical Therapy Science* 28 (7): 2009-13.

Pilates for Chronic Neck Pain

Physiotherapy published a study in 2016 that compared the effectiveness of Pilates and yoga group exercise for pain reduction in individuals with chronic neck pain. The authors pointed out that both methods address the mind–body connection, which is a recognized component in chronic pain management (Lumley et al. 2011), and that there are cost advantages to the group class format used in this study.

In this study, 56 people with chronic neck pain (>3 months) were assigned to one of three groups: control, Pilates, or yoga. The Pilates and yoga groups did 12 small-group sessions over 12 weeks, with modifications and progressions supervised by physiotherapists who had advanced training in that discipline. Outcome measurements were taken prior to the start of classes, at 6 weeks, and at 12 weeks. Follow-up testing was done 6 weeks after completion of the classes. The primary outcome measure was functional ability using the neck disability index questionnaire. Other outcomes tested were pain ratings, range of movement, and postural measurements.

After 12 weeks of weekly group exercise sessions, both the Pilates and yoga groups reported significantly reduced disability and pain compared to a control group; and these improvements were maintained at the 6-week follow-up. Thus the authors concluded that both Pilates and yoga group exercise may be effective and safe short-term methods for addressing chronic neck pain. However, they stressed that these programs must have supervision by qualified professionals, include appropriate modifications, and have a stringent screening process to ensure patients are suitable for group classes.

Dunleavey, K., K. Kava, A. Goldberg, M. H. Malek, S.A. Talley, V. Tutag-Lehr, and J. Hildreth. 2016. Comparative effectiveness of Pilates and yoga group exercise interventions for chronic mechanical neck pain: Quasi-randomised parallel controlled study. *Physiotherapy* 102: 236-42.

Pilates for Prevention of Neck and Shoulder Disorders

A 2010 study looked at the effects of a Pilates program on posture, strength, flexibility, and biomechanical patterns of the neck–shoulder area. Based on previous studies that showed positive effects of Pilates on biomechanical characteristics of spine and lower limb alignment, the authors hypothesized that a 12-week program would improve posture, motion, and arm–trunk muscle patterns.

In the study, 19 healthy subjects were randomly assigned to either an experimental group or a control group and assessed twice: at baseline and after 12 weeks. The assessment consisted of seated posture, abdominal strength, shoulder ROM, and maximal shoulder flexion during which neck, shoulder, and trunk kinematics and the activity of 16 muscles were recorded. The Pilates group did two one-hour private sessions of Pilates per week using the mat, reformer and Cadillac. The control subjects were told not to begin any new physical activity.

After training, subjects in the Pilates group showed smaller thoracic kyphosis during sitting and greater abdominal strength. In addition, these subjects were able to perform the maximal shoulder flexion test with less motion of the shoulder girdle and upper back, suggesting an increased ability to dissociate limb and core motion after Pilates training. The reduced scapular displacements seen indicate an improved ability to stabilize the scapula. Based on several studies that have found that poor thoracic posture, abnormal shoulder biomechanics, and scapular instability are often a cause or effect of neck–shoulder disorders, the results of this study support the hypothesis that Pilates training could help prevent such disorders.

Emery, K., S. J. De Serres, A. McMillan, and J. N. Cote. 2010. The effects of a Pilates training program on arm-trunk posture and movement. *Clinical Biomechanics* 25: 124-30.

Pilates for Treating Rotator Cuff Tendinopathy

A 2016 study by Akbas and Erdem in Turkey set out to determine whether a clinical Pilates exercise program designed specifically for the shoulder muscles is superior to a traditional physiotherapy program in patients with rotator cuff tendinopathy. Referring to the potential benefits of Pilates exercises on connective tissue and overuse injuries that have been reported in the literature (Anderson and Spector 2000; Kloubec 2010), the authors hypothesized that use of Pilates principles and exercises in patients with rotator cuff tendinopathy will yield positive results.

The study included 19 volunteers with a diagnosis of rotator cuff tendinopathy who were randomly assigned to either a Pilates group or a control group. Both groups were treated with hot packs and ultrasound for 15 sessions and were instructed in a home exercise program of traditional wall and wand exercises to strengthen and stretch the upper extremities. In each of the 15 sessions, the

Pilates group also did a supervised 20- to 30-minute Pilates exercise protocol on the mat with a resistance band and a ball according to their abilities.

All patients in the study filled out the following self-report questionnaires at baseline and after three weeks: visual analog scale to assess pain intensity; Disabilities of the Arm, Shoulder and Hand (DASH) and Shoulder Pain and Disability Index (SPADI) to assess disability level; the Stanford Health Assessment Questionnaire and Disability Index (HAQ-DI) to assess general health level; and Beck Anxiety Inventory (BAI) to assess anxiety level. Preintervention scores were similar in both groups. After the three weeks, both groups reported significant decreases in night pain, pain in internal and external rotation, and DASH and SPADI scores. However, only the Pilates group reported decreases in resting pain, pain with flexion and abduction, and HAQ and BAI scores.

The authors pointed out that some improvement was expected in both groups because all patients were receiving physiotherapy treatment. They attributed the less painful movement experienced by patients in the Pilates group to the emphasis placed on the Pilates principles of breathing and concentration during exercise execution (Kloubec 2010). They also felt that diminishing anxiety was an important factor (as evidenced by the lower BAI scores in the Pilates group). It is widely accepted that depression and anxiety are contributory causes for patients with musculoskeletal pain. Pilates is associated with better quality of life values, especially in dimensions of physical functioning, general health, and mental health (Viera et al. 2013). Finally, the authors referred to a 2000 article written by Anderson and Spector which examines how current scientific theories in motor learning and biomechanics relate to the theoretic foundations of the Pilates method. The case was made that Pilates exercises provide a closed-chain environment that facilitates compressive and decompressive forces on the connective tissues, thereby improving circulation. They proposed that this improvement in circulation activated healing mechanisms in the tendons, thus increasing pain-free elevation.

Akbas, E., and E. U. Erdem. 2016. Does Pilates-based approach provide additional benefit over traditional physiotherapy in the management of rotator cuff tendinopathy? A randomized controlled trial. *Annals of Sports Medicine and Research* 3 (6): 1083.

Pilates for the Lower Extremities

Moving down the kinetic chain to the lower extremities, there is much less published research available for review. It is generally agreed upon, however, that the rationale for use of a Pilates program for lower extremity issues is based on the concept of core strengthening (Wilson et al. 2005). One study by Zazulak et al. (2007) measured core neuromuscular control properties of active proprioceptive repositioning and trunk displacement in female collegiate athletes, then tracked their injuries for three years. They found that deficient trunk core stability was a risk factor for anterior cruciate ligament injury. Both this study and other research imply that decreased core stability may predispose one to lower extremity injuries and suggest that achieving core stability is crucial to establishing a stable base for movement of the extremities. Pilates, then, which has been shown to improve core strength (Emery et al. 2010; Kloubec 2010), is an ideal exercise modality for treatment and prevention of lower extremity injuries.

Pilates Research Review: The Lower Extremities

Pilates for Total Hip or Total Knee Arthroplasty

Orthopedic surgeons William Jaffe and Brett Levine, along with registered nurse and Pilates instructor Beth Kaplanek, developed a specific Pilates protocol for patients to follow after total hip or total knee arthroplasty. The authors touted Pilates as an integrative approach for a complete body workout that can be easily modified depending on the individual limitations and surgeon-based restrictions. Patients who expressed interest in Pilates were encouraged to start training preoperatively with a certified Pilates instructor and to begin the postoperative program within two weeks of discharge from the hospital. They prescribed a specific set of modified Pilates mat exercises for both the total hip replacement and total knee replacement patients to be performed a minimum of three to four times per week for at least one hour.

After one year, a group of 38 patients including 30 women and 8 men (21 total hip arthroplasties and 17 total knee arthroplasties) who followed the prescribed Pilates protocol were followed up with via chart notes and phone calls and reported the following results: 25 were extremely satisfied, 13 were satisfied, and 0 were somewhat satisfied or not satisfied. Most of the women in the study (73 percent) reported continuing with Pilates on a routine basis.

In addition, the senior author reported using Pilates with his patients for the prior five years without a single negative event and with a high degree of patient satisfaction, both physically and emotionally. This is a preliminary report on a small sample of patients and, as such, it did not set out to prove that Pilates is better than traditional therapy, but to offer Pilates as a viable option for rehabilitation after total hip and knee arthroplasty.

Levine B., B. Kaplanek, and W. L. Jaffe. 2009. Pilates training for use in rehabilitation after total hip and knee arthroplasty: A preliminary report. *Clinical Orthopaedics and Related Research* 467: 1468-75.

Pilates After Total Hip Arthroplasty

In 2007, Klein et al. developed a web-based survey to evaluate joint arthroplasty surgeons' preferences for the return to sporting activities after total hip arthroplasty. This survey listed 30 groups of activities (37 specific sports) and was sent to all members of the Hip Society and the American Association of Hip and Knee Surgeons. Pilates was rated as a sports activity that patients are allowed to participate in after a total hip arthroplasty. However, surgeons take Pilates experience into consideration; 58 percent of the surgeons surveyed allowed their post-op patients to participate in Pilates without previous experience, and an additional 24 percent recommended to allow participation only for those with previous experience.

Klein, G. R., B. R. Levine, W. J. Hozack, E. J. Strausse, J. A. D'Antonio, W. Macaulay, and P. E. Di Cesare. 2007. Return to athletic activity after total hip arthroplasty. Consensus guidelines based on a survey of the Hip Society and American Association of Hip and Knee Surgeons. *Journal of Arthroplasty* 22: 171-75.

Pilates for Partial Anterior Cruciate Ligament (ACL) Tears

A 2017 study by Celik and Turkel looked at the effects of Pilates on muscle strength, function, and knee instability for patients with a partial ACL tear in which nonsurgical treatment was preferred. Fifty participants between 20 and 45 years of age were randomly assigned to either the Pilates exercise group or the control group. The authors designed a specific program of basic Pilates mat exercises focused on core stability and lower extremity strength and flexibility. The Pilates group participated in a 60-minute group class three times per week for 12 weeks. The control group did not receive any treatment or a home exercise program. Functional scores and isokinetic strength were assessed at baseline and at the end of the 12 weeks by a physical therapist.

Per quadriceps strength testing, the Pilates group experienced significant improvement over that of the control group. Though both groups showed improvement in knee function (assessed via the Lysholm Knee Scoring Scale and the Cincinnati Knee Rating System), the Pilates group's results were of a larger magnitude. According to the responses of the patients in the Pilates group on the global rating of change scale, 88 percent stated that they felt much better in terms of stability, and 12 percent reported they were slightly better. The authors believed that the decreased feelings of the knee giving way reported by the Pilates group were due to improved core strength. In the control group, only 23 percent reported to be slightly better, 38 percent felt the same, and 38 percent said they had deteriorated slightly.

This study concluded that participation in Pilates resulted in superior recovery when compared to no exercise participation. The authors suggested that because Pilates was shown to improve quadriceps strength and subjectively increase both knee stability and function, it may provide clinicians a novel option when choosing a treatment for a partial anterior cruciate ligament injury.

Celik, D., and N. Turkel. 2017. The effectiveness of Pilates for partial anterior cruciate ligament injury. *Knee Surgery, Sports Traumatology, Arthroscopy* 25 (8): 2357-64.

Case Study: Pilates for Recurrent Lower Extremity Injuries

Current Sports Medicine Reports published an interesting case study of a 48-year-old high-level female runner with 25 years of recurrent lower extremity injuries. The athlete's injuries included patellofemoral pain syndrome, iliotibial band syndrome, plantar fasciitis, groin pain, sacroiliac joint dysfunction, and eventually an inability to run due to falls from catching her right foot. Over a span of 20 years, she had numerous diagnostic tests to determine the cause of these issues, but no definitive explanation was found. Thus she was given the diagnosis of proximal instability and dysfunction of the hip, spine, and pelvic stabilizers that resulted in lower extremity malalignment and a disabling movement pattern. At the time of this study she had been unable to run for three years despite trying multiple treatment approaches, including an orthotics prescription, cortisone injections, NSAIDs, manual physical therapy, and leg-strengthening exercises using both elastic bands and weights.

Upon physical therapy evaluation by the authors, the patient was found to have weak hip abductors and external rotators, a typical pattern seen in distance runners due to working primarily in the sagittal plane. To treat this, they designed a Pilates-evolved functional movement protocol with the goal of improving control and strength of the proximal stabilizers through all planes of motion. After one year of this program (two days per week of 60- to 90-minute sessions and a home exercise program), her disabling movement pattern resolved, and she returned to regular running. Thus, the Pilates-based exercise program resolved this runner's lower extremity malalignment and returned her to running when other traditional treatment approaches did not.

Lugo-Larcheveque N., L. S. Pescatello, T. W. Dugdale, D. M. Veltri, and W. O. Roberts. 2006. Management of lower extremity malalignment during running with neuromuscular retraining of the proximal stabilizers. *Current Sports Medicine Reports* 5 (3): 137-40.

The research studies reviewed in this chapter provide evidence that Pilates is indeed effective in injury rehab, and even prehab. Studies like these go a long way in helping to establish the case for the use of Pilates in physiotherapy and athletic training. Although there is not an overwhelming amount of research on Pilates specifically for injury rehab, it is both encouraging and exciting to see more being published each year. As more scientific studies are conducted, I am confident that Pilates will continue to gain respect as a modality that offers not just conditioning and core strength benefits, but a myriad of other advantages for orthopedic injuries.

As someone who has used Pilates exercises and principles to rehabilitate numerous patients for many years, I have always believed that the excellent outcomes achieved are associated with increased core strength and enhanced mind–body connection. The next chapter discusses the guiding principles of Pilates and delves further into this concept of mind–body connection. It is widely accepted that these principles are what make Pilates a mind–body form of conditioning rather than only a physical process.

2

Guiding Principles of Pilates

Physical fitness is the first requisite of happiness. Our interpretation of physical fitness is the maintenance of a uniformly developed body with a sound mind fully capable of naturally, easily, and satisfactorily performing our many and varied daily tasks with spontaneous zest and pleasure (Pilates 1945, 15).

In Joseph Pilates' book, *Return to Life Through Contrology*, he writes that his method is not merely a physical fitness regimen of mindlessly repeated exercises, but rather a holistic approach to well-being and a lifelong process of refinement. Besides describing his exercises, he gives advice on many things: optimal sleeping conditions, the importance of getting plenty of sunshine and fresh air, proper diet and the detriment of overeating for your activity level, appropriate attire for exercise, standing and walking techniques, and even how to really achieve thorough cleanliness with showering methods. He makes some bold statements, but his philosophy is consistent: the mind, body, and spirit are intricately linked.

Contrology is complete coordination of body, mind, and spirit. Contrology develops the body uniformly, corrects wrong postures, restores physical vitality, invigorates the mind, and elevates the spirit (Pilates 1945, 18).

An in-depth exploration of each aspect of Pilates' method, which he called "contrology," would far exceed the parameters of this book. Our focus is on the rehab and prehab benefits of Pilates, with the goal of demonstrating movements and postures that help an athlete improve performance, reduce the risk of further injury, and maximize training after effectively healing from an injury. However, to not address the classic principles of the method would be unjust.

Depending on the school of Pilates, the guiding principles and the way in which they are presented may vary slightly; however, it is widely accepted that some version of these principles are what make Pilates a mind–body form of conditioning rather than only a physical process. I feel it is important to introduce the principles as they were taught to me by my teacher, Rael Isacowitz, in the Body Arts and Science International (BASI) Pilates teacher training program. In addition, I have added my thoughts on their relation to physiotherapy in clinical practice over the years.

Three Higher Principles

1. Completely coordinate the body, mind, and spirit.
2. Achieve the natural inner rhythm associated with all subconscious activities.
3. Apply the natural laws of life to everyday living.

In Isacowitz's book, *Pilates*, he summarizes three themes, which he calls the higher principles of the method. He points out that as new research is conducted and modern technology created, certain elements of the work and the way in which we describe or perform the movements may change, but "the philosophy encompassed in these three principles never changes ... It is the essence of the system itself" (Isacowitz 2014, 5).

From these higher principles, Isacowitz has identified 10 movement principles that form the foundation of the BASI Pilates method. These principles are an amalgamation of those cited in the writings and teachings of Joseph Pilates and those that have evolved from over 40 years of Isacowitz's experience in practice and teaching. It is these principles that make the Pilates method unique and differentiate it from other forms of conditioning. Isacowitz emphasizes that to truly reap the benefits of this method, we must keep all of these principles in mind when both practicing and teaching it to others.

The 10 Principles of BASI Pilates

1. Awareness
2. Balance
3. Breath
4. Concentration
5. Center
6. Control
7. Efficiency
8. Flow
9. Precision
10. Harmony

Awareness

Pilates is practiced in an environment that stimulates the mind–body connection, beginning with an awareness of the body. (Isacowitz 2014, 6)

Without awareness, change cannot occur. We all develop postural misalignments, incorrect movement patterns, and compensations over time. If we are not aware of these, how can we correct them? The less aware a person is, the more severe these issues can become. Often I will be working with a patient in supine on the reformer and I will notice that his hips are shifted a few inches (several centimeters) to the left. When I ask him to straighten out his body, the reply is, "I am straight." If I allow this patient to continue to think that crooked is straight, how are we ever going to achieve correct alignment, muscular balance, and proper movement? How is his injury ever going to heal?

Balance

You should strive to achieve balance, in every sense of the word, and make it an integral part of your Pilates practice. (Isacowitz 2014, 6)

The principle of achieving balance in Pilates means many things. As a physical therapist, when I hear the term *balance* I think of whether or not a patient can stand on one leg with the eyes closed or what his score will be on the Berg Balance Scale. Although Pilates does help with this type of balance, we are also referring to a balanced program in which both stability and mobility are addressed, as well as ensuring that all areas of the body are worked. Additionally, the balance or well-being of the whole person (body, mind, and spirit) is considered.

In the rehabilitation realm, however, I most often apply this principle to the symmetry of the body. Musculoskeletal conditions frequently show patterns of imbalance. Some are associated with simple side dominance or handedness, as most of us have a stronger side and a weaker side. Imbalances are also created by recreational and occupational positions and movements. Movement habits in which certain muscles are recruited excessively while others are underutilized are created. An example we see all too often in the modern world is someone who sits at a desk all day. The patient will often present with tight, overactive hip flexors but inactive, weak gluteal muscles. Often imbalances are caused by the body using compensatory mechanisms to protect certain areas or to reduce pain, resulting in facilitation of some muscles and inhibition of others. For example, a patient with a rotator cuff tear in the shoulder frequently develops a tight upper trapezius and levator scapulae. Each person has unique imbalances, and these are almost always related to their injury or dysfunctional pattern. Identifying and addressing these imbalances and figuring out how to alleviate them is the first step back to wellness.

Breath

Breathing is synonymous with life and with movement. It is all-encompassing: the link between body, mind, and spirit ... it is the engine that drives all movement, and it lies at the source of the Pilates method. (Isacowitz 2014, 7)

Breathing is the first act of life, and the last. Our very life depends on it. Lazy breathing converts the lungs, figuratively speaking, into a cemetery for the deposition of diseased, dying, and dead germs. (Pilates 1945, 23)

Besides keeping us alive, breathing has many physiological advantages, including the following:

- Oxygenates the blood
- Releases toxins
- Improves circulation
- Calms the mind and body
- Facilitates concentration
- Provides a rhythm for movement
- Assists in activating target muscles

For all of these reasons, correct breathing is very important in Pilates and in rehabilitation to achieve optimal results.

Natural or diaphragmatic breathing encourages relaxation of the abdominal muscles during inhalation. In Pilates, lateral or intercostal breathing is used. With this type of breathing, an effort is made to emphasize the lateral and posterior expansion of the rib cage during inhalation, which promotes a consistent inward pull of the abdominal wall. As accessory muscles of exhalation, the abdominals contract more during this phase of breathing to assist the diaphragm and intercostal muscles in expelling air. Thus, with lateral breathing, the maintenance of abdominal muscle contraction is facilitated throughout the breathing cycle, which in turn helps stabilize the trunk (see figure 2.1).

It is widely accepted by Pilates professionals that the use of breath has significant importance in the practice of the method; however, there are often disagreements as to whether a particular breath pattern is best. In BASI Pilates, the basic breath pattern used is to exhale with spinal flexion and inhale with spinal extension. Why? Besides providing a natural rhythm for the movements, the abdominals are trunk flexors as well as accessory muscles in exhalation. The TrA, in particular, has been shown to be recruited first and to have a lower threshold for recruitment during active exhalation (Abe et al. 1996; De Troyer et al. 1990; Hodges and Gandavia 2000). As was discussed in chapter 1, the TrA is one of the key muscles in spinal stabilization. So theoretically, if an exhalation during

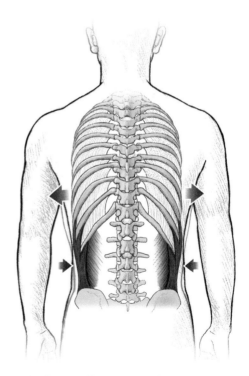

FIGURE 2.1 Expansion of the rib cage during inhalation when using lateral breathing.

spinal flexion maximizes activation of the TrA, we are maximizing trunk stability. Following with this reasoning, studies have shown that the latissimus dorsi is an accessory muscle in inhalation (Cala, Edyvean, and Engel 1992; Orozco-Levi et al. 1995), so we can maximize activation of the spinal extensors when actively inhaling. In exercises where we are not specifically flexing or extending the spine, the breath pattern is to exhale on the effort.

Although classically there is an emphasis on set breathing technique, often when working with patients I have found that too much emphasis on correct breathing can be counterproductive. Some functional movement patterns require timing that can be disrupted if too much focus is placed on breathing. And many patients are already challenged enough—dealing with an injury and learning new movements—so having to think about breathing as well can make for a frustrating experience. Too much emphasis on the breath pattern makes it difficult or even impossible to focus on the technique, thereby decreasing the neuromuscular reeducational benefits of the exercise. So quite often, the first priority is learning to execute the movement safely and correctly, and the breathing pattern is introduced later.

Concentration

I view concentration as the bridge between awareness and movement. (Isacowitz 2014, 9)

Always keep your mind wholly concentrated on the purpose of the exercises as you perform them. This is vitally important in order for you to gain the results sought. (Pilates 1945, 20)

Due to the mind–body connection, simply tapping into or concentrating on a particular muscle or muscle group can result in more accurate and intense activation of it. For Pilates exercises to be effective, it is important to concentrate not only on the recruitment of specific muscles, but also on correct body alignment. Focusing on maintaining correct alignment and stabilization throughout the exercises ensures recruitment of the proper muscle groups for the desired action and avoids unnecessary strain. In many circumstances, concentrating on the breathing pattern helps maintain rhythm for the movement and keeps the mind focused. In Pilates, however, we do not want the concentration to be so intense that it causes tightening of the muscles or restriction of breathing. This would be counterproductive to what we are trying to achieve.

Center

In Pilates, centering yourself means more than finding your center of gravity; it means uniting body, mind, and spirit. (Isacowitz 2014, 9)

Physically speaking, finding one's center refers simply to the place in one's body that is one's center of gravity. This will be slightly different for each individual, based on his or her specific anatomy. But in Pilates, the word *center* means much more. The concept that all movement originates from the center or core is a common theme in Pilates. It is often termed the *powerhouse* in Pilates; it is described by Isacowitz as the internal support system; and it is sometimes referred to as the local muscle system in the rehabilitation realm (see figure 2.2). Whichever term you prefer, we are talking about the deep, intrinsic muscles of the trunk. These transversus abdominis, multifidi, diaphragm, and pelvic floor muscles attach directly to the spine and offer stabilization. Note that none of these muscles can be easily accessed, as they are deep lying and are not developed in the same way that other skeletal muscles are, such as the biceps or quadriceps. Perhaps this is why the mind–body approach of Pilates works so well in spinal stabilization; it allows us to get deeper and facilitates this neuromuscular connection.

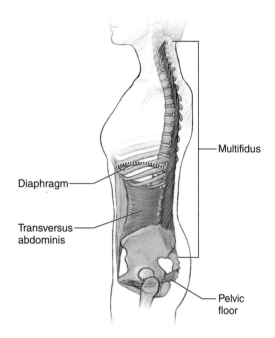

FIGURE 2.2 The local muscle system or internal support system.

Control

Contrology begins with mind control over muscles. (Pilates 1945, 19)

Refining control is inherent in mastering a skill. Refined control requires a great deal of practice, which can aid in developing the necessary strength and flexibility of key muscles as well as allow for the development of more refined motor programs. (Isacowitz and Clippinger 2011, 2)

Initially, gaining control of our movements is a conscious process, and it takes a lot of practice. However, once mastered, it can become innate. Think of an Olympic sprinter versus a child learning to walk. The athlete clearly has a higher level of control than the child, and thus a lower risk of injury. Learning which muscles are needed to control our movements and being able to maintain control throughout the exercises is an important concept in Pilates. Flailing about is not allowed. Neither momentum nor brute force—but rather precise neuromuscular control of the appropriate muscles—is used to achieve a movement.

Efficiency

When performing Pilates we do not grimace during effort, nor grunt as the movements become difficult and demanding. We focus the work where it is needed, exerting the required amount of energy, no more and no less. (Isacowitz 2014, 10)

This Pilates principle teaches us to conserve energy and to use only the necessary muscles to achieve the functional task or goal. Inefficiency in our movement patterns is counterproductive to the functional task and can lead to less-than-stellar results as well as imbalances, pain, and injuries. Take a golf swing, for example. Studies show that professional golfers have 50 percent less electromyogram activity than an amateur. What they have mastered is a highly refined movement, which requires efficient muscular activity (Donatelli 2009).

Flow

As do all of the principles in Pilates, *flow* has both physical and mental connotations. In positive psychology, it is defined by psychologist Mihaly Csikszentmihalyi as "being completely involved in an activity for its own sake. The ego falls away. Time flies. Every action, movement, and thought follows inevitably from the previous one, like playing jazz. Your whole being is involved, and you're using your skills to the utmost"(Gierland 1996). It is similar to being in the zone.

Physiologically, flow can be understood as "the immaculate timing of muscle recruitment" (Isacowitz 2014, 11), or what we call the muscle firing or muscle activation sequence. For each movement, there is an optimal sequence in which the muscles should fire. When this is not followed, tightness or pain is often experienced because certain muscles become overused and tight. In injury rehabilitation, it is important to restore the correct muscle firing sequence, or *flow*. Both the physical and the mental aspects of flow are demonstrated beautifully in athletes such as Michael Phelps or Simone Biles. They make supremely difficult movements appear effortless. This is what we strive for and what can be achieved by practicing Pilates.

Precision

The greater the precision, the more likely the goal will be achieved and the greater the benefit from doing the exercise. (Isacowitz and Clippinger 2011, 2)

Precision is one of the most obvious differences between Pilates and other types of exercise. Similar to how yoga becomes just like calisthenics when done without deep breathing and mindfulness, without precision, Pilates exercises become almost meaningless.

Precision can be defined as the exact manner in which an action is executed. Many of the Pilates exercises themselves are not so different from the traditional versions learned in physiotherapy school, but the way in which they are executed is very different. Take, for example, the chest lift exercise (p. 61). The actual movement may appear to be the same as an abdominal crunch or a sit-up. In a gym or boot camp we see people doing hundreds of repetitions without apparent fatigue, using many muscles and momentum to achieve the movement. However, my patients and clients often comment that they feel it in the abs more than ever after just a few repetitions due to the precision with which the Pilates chest lift is executed. Complete muscle integration, which is often followed by the isolation of certain muscles or muscle groups, is required to achieve precision. The work is felt more profoundly and is more effective when every movement is executed with precision.

Harmony

Harmony is the whole, the culmination of all we strive to achieve. It means being focused, centered, and in control, moving efficiently coupled with flow and precision. (Isacowitz 2014, 12)

The way in which one interprets and integrates these principles into the practice of Pilates will vary. To those of us with a medical or scientific background, the physical aspects of these principles will be emphasized as we use Pilates to rehabilitate injuries and enhance athletic performance. For others (perhaps our clients or patients), the mental aspects will resonate with them and will allow them to reach a greater potential. But either way, the important thing to understand is that Pilates is not simply exercise; it is a holistic approach to optimizing human movement. To truly reap the benefits of this method, we must keep all of these principles in mind when both practicing and teaching it to others.

I have seen numerous patients over the years reach a far greater potential when the mental aspect of these principles is integrated into the motor learning and neuromuscular reeducation process. When I give traditional home exercise programs to patients, it is rare that they continue doing them after (or even during) their prescribed injury rehab. However, patients often enjoy the Pilates exercises and feel the benefits so much that they continue with Pilates, enrolling in ongoing private sessions or group classes. Thus, I have not only rehabilitated their injury, but I have also introduced them to a new form of exercise and encouraged them to maintain a healthy lifestyle.

3

Integrating Pilates With Rehabilitation

Chapters 1 and 2 discussed the principles upon which the Pilates method is based and reviewed research supporting its use in physiotherapy. This chapter will explain why Pilates is so effective—not only to rehabilitate and heal injuries but also to increase overall fitness level, improve performance, or provide safe and effective cross-training in the off-season. But first, I'd like to share with you how and when I discovered Pilates and began integrating it into my practice.

Prior to my career as a physical therapist (PT) I was an exercise instructor for many years, so I had heard of Pilates, but besides a mat class or two I had very little experience with it. While working at Rancho La Puerta Spas just before starting physical therapy school, I had the good fortune of meeting Rael Isacowitz, the founder of BASI Pilates. I remember him telling me it would be a great idea for me to learn Pilates because it is so effective for injury rehab. But my goal was very clear; I wanted to specialize in orthopedics and sports medicine and work with athletes. This Pilates stuff was for dancers, right?

A few years later I was working as the PT for the Phoenix Suns basketball team when our star point guard broke his ankle. As he was recovering from surgery, his wife, already a Pilates practitioner, asked me if I had any experience with Pilates. They had a reformer at home, and she thought it would be great if we could use it to help rehab his ankle. I quickly found a Pilates studio and took a session. I was amazed! So many different exercises could be done on one piece of equipment, and it was immediately clear to me how adaptable and appropriate these exercises could be for rehab purposes.

It was then that I decided I needed to be properly trained in the Pilates method. Luckily for me, I had already met my teacher. Isacowitz is one of the most respected professionals in the Pilates industry and recognized worldwide, and BASI Pilates had already been providing top-level comprehensive Pilates education for over 20 years. So I moved back to California, studied and trained with Rael at his studio in Newport Beach, and soon after began integrating Pilates into patient treatments. This was more than 17 years ago, and we have been utilizing Pilates as a treatment modality at our physical therapy and wellness center with excellent patient outcomes ever since.

Why Pilates Works in Injury Rehab and Prevention

Pilates is a great tool to assist or even enhance a physiotherapy program when someone is recovering from an injury. By strengthening the deepest muscles of the core, optimizing alignment, and creating correct movement patterns, we can also help to prevent reaggravation of those injuries and the development of new ones. PTs are always searching for a system that can take patients from the early stages of rehabilitation to the long-term goal of a conditioned, efficiently functioning body. Pilates is that system! Other rehabilitation professionals often ask me, why do you think Pilates works so well in injury rehab and prevention? Here are what I see as the 10 fundamental reasons, both scientific and practical, that Pilates is so effective in injury rehab and prevention.

1. Pilates Focuses on the Center or Core Muscles

As discussed in chapter 2, the core is often referred to as the powerhouse or the internal support system in Pilates, and as the local muscle system in the rehabilitation realm. Whichever term you prefer, we are talking about the deepest intrinsic muscles of the trunk that attach directly to the spine and offer stabilization: transversus abdominis, multifidi, pelvic floor, and diaphragm. The importance of these deep muscles in rehabilitation, primarily for patients with lumbar pathologies, has been well established both in the literature and in clinical practice. However, the term *core strength* is often tagged onto every possible workout routine, resulting in some ambiguity in its meaning.

---

10 Fundamental Reasons Why Pilates is Effective in Injury Rehabilitation and Prevention

1. Pilates focuses on the center or core muscles.
2. Pilates exercises emphasize both stability and mobility.
3. Pilates includes both closed-kinetic-chain and open-kinetic-chain exercises.
4. Pilates exercises work muscles statically and dynamically—emphasizing both concentric and eccentric muscular contractions.
5. Pilates exercises are functional.
6. Pilates places an importance on breathing appropriately.
7. Pilates is adaptable for many different patient populations.
8. Pilates is a mind–body form of conditioning.
9. Pilates equipment is safe and easy to use (with proper training).
10. Pilates is a wise business choice to expand your wellness services.

The BASI Pilates method defines core strength as

> *the strength of the muscles that support the pelvic-lumbar region, and the ability of them to work synergistically, in an integrated and efficient way. It is the functional strength of the deepest, intrinsic muscles of the trunk; those muscles that support the spine, and offer stabilization and movement emanating from the core of the body. (Isacowitz 2006, 1)*

This concept that all movement originates from the center or core is a common theme in Pilates, and much emphasis is placed on recruiting the core muscles for many, if not all of the exercises. Movement is of course possible without activating the internal support system; however, internal support, protection, and efficient function will not be present (Isacowitz 2014).

Abdominals—Transversus Abdominis

The four layers of abdominal muscles, from superficial to deep, are rectus abdominis, external obliques, internal obliques, and transversus abdominis (TrA). All of these muscles are involved in providing stability and strength of the core. However, the muscle that has been established as the most important in terms of spinal support or stabilization is the TrA.

The TrA runs from the rib cage to the pubis, and its fibers are oriented horizontally. It wraps around the entire abdominal cavity and attaches posteriorly to the thoracolumbar fascia like a girdle. When the TrA contracts, it pulls the abdominal wall inward, compressing the abdominal cavity and thus providing lumbo-pelvic stability. This muscle does not move any joints, so it can be difficult to recruit or isolate (see figure 3.1).

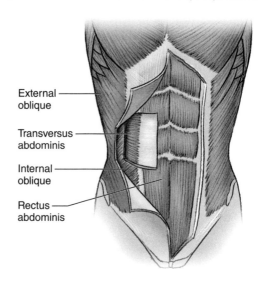

External oblique

Transversus abdominis

Internal oblique

Rectus abdominis

FIGURE 3.1 The abdominal muscles.

Back Extensors—Multifidi

Arranged in layers similar to the abdominal muscles, the back extensors include the erector spinae, semispinalis, and deep posterior groups (see figure 3.2). All of these muscles are involved in providing strength and stability to the core, but the muscles that can be singled out in terms of spinal stabilization are the multifidi, part of the deep posterior group. Each multifidus spans two to three joint segments and functions to stabilize the vertebrae at each segmental level. This local segmental stability makes each vertebra work more effectively, thus reducing degeneration of the joints. Dysfunction of the multifidus has been demonstrated in patients with low back pain as compared to normal subjects. Differences are seen in muscle activation patterns, fatigability, muscle composition, and muscle size and consistency (Richardson, Jull, and

Hodges 2004). Research has established that during an abdominal drawing in maneuver, the multifidus muscle cocontracts with the TrA (Richardson, Jull, and Hodges, 2004). Hides et al. (2011) showed clinically that the ability to contract the multifidus muscle is related to the ability to contract the TrA, with the odds of a good contraction of multifidus being four and a half times higher for those who have a good contraction of TrA.

Pelvic Floor Muscles

The pelvic floor muscles consist of the levator ani group (iliococcygeus, pubococcygeus, and puborectalis) and the coccygeus. They provide a sling of support for the inner viscera and adapt to the changes in internal pressure of the abdominal cavity (see figure 3.3). When they are recruited, they increase intra-abdominal pressure, thereby unloading the spine. Electromyogram studies by Sapsford et al. (2001) have shown that activation of the TrA is neurophysiologically linked to the activation of the pelvic floor muscles. Abdominal muscle activity is a normal response to pelvic floor exercise (in subjects without pelvic floor muscle dysfunction) and conversely, submaximal isometric abdominal exercises activate the pelvic floor muscles.

Diaphragm

The diaphragm, a respiratory muscle responsible for drawing air into the lungs, forms the lid of the internal support system (see figure 3.4). Research by Hodges and Gandevia (2000) showed that coactivation of the diaphragm and abdominal muscles causes a sustained increase in intra-abdominal pressure. Thus, the diaphragm assists in the mechanical stabilization of the spine in conjunction with contraction of the abdominal and pelvic floor muscles (Kolar et al. 2012).

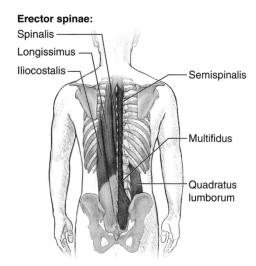

FIGURE 3.2 The back extensors.

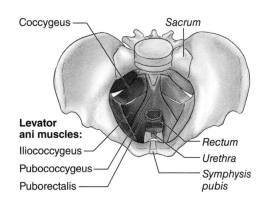

FIGURE 3.3 The muscles of the pelvic floor.

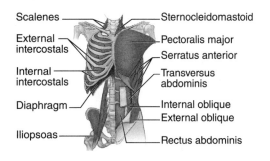

FIGURE 3.4 The muscles of the diaphragm.

Muscles of the Upper Core

So far we have talked about the importance of core strength only in relation to the lower spine. But core strength is important in the upper spine as well. Many people exhibit forward head and rounded shoulder posture associated with muscle imbalances and often neck pain. For these patients, it is important to take it one more step and consider what I call the upper core: deep neck flexors (DNFs), lower trapezius, and serratus anterior.

Many years ago, Dr. Vladamir Janda referred to the specific patterns of muscle imbalance often seen in patients with cervical dysfunction *upper crossed syndrome* (Page, Frank, and Lardner 2010). The specific postural changes seen in this type of syndrome include forward head posture, increased cervical lordosis and thoracic kyphosis, elevated and protracted shoulders, and rotation or abduction and winging of the scapulae (Page 2011). In order to help a patient with this type of syndrome, we must address the muscle imbalances and correct the faulty posture (see figure 3.5).

Based on the clinical teachings of Dr. Janda, one of the areas where these patients have marked weakness or muscular inhibition is the deep neck flexors (longus colli and longus capitis). Research by Jull, O'Leary, and Falla (2008) confirmed that neck pain patients have an altered neuromotor control strategy during craniocervical flexion characterized by reduced activity in the deep cervical flexors and increased activity in the superficial flexors (SCM and anterior scalene muscles). Their studies indicate that this impairment is generic to neck pain disorders, regardless of the specific pathology. As established through this and subsequent research, training of the deep neck flexors is effective at reducing neck pain symptoms. Widely used in clinical practice, this neuromuscular retraining is accomplished via isolated upper cervical spine flexion: a gentle nodding motion with the chin (often referred to as a chin nod or chin tuck) followed by a 10 second isometric hold without activating the SCM or scalene muscles (see Chapter 4, p. 43).

In addition to the inhibition and weakness of the deep neck flexors, several studies point to poor thoracic posture, abnormal shoulder biomechanics, and scapular instability as a cause or effect of neck–shoulder disorders (Emery et al. 2010). Stability around the shoulder blades is crucial for efficient movement of the arms and neck. While there are many muscles involved in stabilizing the scapula, the main stabilizers are the serratus anterior, rhomboids, levator scapulae, and trapezius. Imbalances in these muscles can lead to abnormal positioning of the scapula, disturbances in scapulohumeral rhythm, and generalized shoulder complex dysfunction (Kamkar, Irrgang, and Whitney 1993).

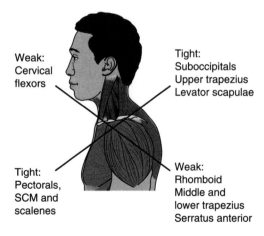

Weak:
Cervical flexors

Tight:
Suboccipitals
Upper trapezius
Levator scapulae

Tight:
Pectorals,
SCM and
scalenes

Weak:
Rhomboid
Middle and
lower trapezius
Serratus anterior

FIGURE 3.5 Upper crossed syndrome.

A common issue seen in people with neck or shoulder pain is excessive elevation of the scapula when raising the arm. Thus, strength and proper functioning of the scapular depressors, lower trapezius, and serratus anterior is key (see figure 3.6). Consistent with Janda's upper crossed syndrome theory, more recent research has shown that the serratus anterior and lower trapezius are the most commonly weak or inhibited muscles of the scapulothoracic joint that may lead to this abnormal movement (Paine and Voight 2013).

It is interesting to note that none of these internal support system muscles can be easily accessed as they are deep lying. Thus recruiting and isolating them is difficult, requiring mental focus, awareness, and concentration. These deep muscles also cannot be developed in the same way as other skeletal muscles such as the biceps or quadriceps. Perhaps this is why the mind–body approach of Pilates works so well in spinal stabilization and rehabilitation; it allows us to get deeper and facilitates this difficult-to-achieve neuromuscular connection. Recent research points to a motor control rather than a pure strength perspective in the management of pain and indicates that impaired neuromotor control does not recover automatically even with resolution of pain. Specific retraining is required (Hides et al. 1996; Jull et al. 2002). Thus, the neuromuscular development of these deep muscles that can be achieved through Pilates principles and exercises serves as the foundation on which true, functional, core strength can be built.

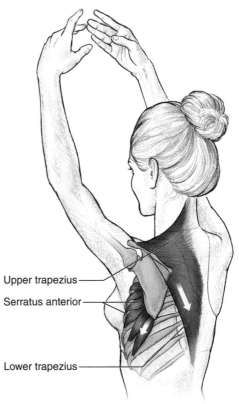

Upper trapezius

Serratus anterior

Lower trapezius

FIGURE 3.6 Strength and proper functioning of the scapular depressors is necessary to prevent excessive elevation of the scapulae when raising the arms overhead.

As small bricks are employed to build large buildings, so will the development of small muscles help develop large muscles. (Pilates 1945, 25)

2. Pilates Exercises Emphasize Both Stability and Mobility

A strong, optimally functioning body must be both stable and mobile. Adequate stabilization proximally enables us to attain optimal function distally. Take, for example, a tennis player: he must have proximal strength and stability of his shoulder girdle, yet tremendous mobility in the arm to be able to efficiently hit the ball. If the shoulder is weak or unstable it is likely that an injury will occur over time. The common tennis injury lateral epicondylitis, or tennis elbow, is often caused by late strokes and "wristy" impact due to a lack of scapular stability, which places too much stress on the elbow and wrist joints. One of the ways we treat this is to strengthen the muscles of the arm, shoulder, and upper back to help take stress off of the elbow. Can we do this with Pilates exercises? Absolutely! However, if the shoulder girdle is so stable that it doesn't move, it is not possible to raise the arm overhead into the proper position to deliver a powerful serve. Thus, exercises that mobilize the shoulder complex are also important, and there are many of these in the Pilates repertoire as well.

Being too loose (hypermobility) or too tight (hypomobility) can both lead to injuries and pathologies. Weight-lifting regimens often emphasize stability to the point where the person is so stable he or she cannot move. Certain types of yoga or stretching programs, on the other hand, focus so much on stretching that people end up with a weak core and hyperflexibility, which can lead to conditions of instability.

In Pilates, some of the exercises focus on stability (front support, p. 74), some focus on mobility (kneeling arm circles, p. 134) and many provide a perfect combination of both (diagonal pull p. 131). Thus, Pilates emphasizes both stability and mobility, allowing us to achieve optimal performance and helping to prevent injuries.

Stability + Mobility = Agility. (Brourman, 2010)

3. Pilates Includes Both Closed-Kinetic-Chain and Open-Kinetic-Chain Exercises

An open-kinetic-chain exercise is one in which the distal segment (hand or foot) moves freely in space, such as a biceps curl with a free weight or a prone hamstrings curl using a resistance band. In Pilates there are many open-chain exercises: single-leg side series—circles (p. 180), arms supine series (beginning on p. 97), and hip work series (beginning on p. 108), to name a few. Open-chain exercises are wonderful for increasing joint mobility and for conditions such as osteoarthritis, in which strengthening the muscles in a non–weight-bearing position is important.

A closed-kinetic-chain exercise is one in which the distal segment is fixed and cannot move. The hand or foot remains in constant contact with a surface, usually the ground or the base of a machine. A classic example of a closed-chain exercise for the upper extremity is a push-up (called front support in Pilates, p. 74). For the lower extremity, a traditional example is a squat or leg press. In the Pilates repertoire, there are many closed-chain exercises. For example: footwork (p. 88), standing leg press (p. 212), and backward step-down (p. 216). Because closed-chain exercises require cocontraction of the muscles surrounding the joint, they promote joint stability. Therefore, closed-chain exercises are recommended for conditions of instability—for example, an ankle sprain or a shoulder subluxation. The fact that closed-chain exercises are weight-bearing makes them very useful for pathologies such as osteoporosis, in which load helps to rebuild bone mass.

Functionally, most of our activities of daily living are both open and closed chain. Walking, for example, is closed-chain on the stance leg but open-chain on the swing leg. Pilates exercises such as scooter (p. 155) and standing leg press (p. 212) simulate this type of action, making them very functional types of exercise. The concept of functionality is an important one in rehabilitation and will be discussed in more detail later in this chapter.

4. Pilates Exercises Work Muscles Statically and Dynamically—Emphasizing Both Concentric and Eccentric Muscular Contractions

A static or isometric contraction is one in which there is no visible change in muscle length nor observable joint movement. Although the muscle is generating tension, the effect of the muscle contraction is exactly counterbalanced by the effect of the resistance, resulting in no net movement (Isacowitz and Clippinger 2011). Typically the body's stabilizing muscles (TrA, for example) function isometrically.

An isotonic or dynamic contraction is one in which the muscle contracts through a range of motion against a resistive force. The length of the muscle and the angle of the joint changes. A concentric contraction is considered a positive movement; the muscle shortens, and the angle of the joint decreases. An eccentric contraction involves lengthening of the muscle (the distance between the attachment points becomes greater) with movement in the direction opposite to that of the action of the primary muscle. An eccentric contraction is used as a means of decelerating a body part or object, or lowering a load gently rather than letting it drop. Heavy eccentric loading results in greater muscular damage, and often, delayed onset muscle soreness occurs one to two days after training. Eccentric training has been shown to be a successful intervention for postrehabilitation injury recovery, especially for lower body injuries (Alfredson and Lorentzon 2000; Bahr et al. 2006; Mafi et al. 2001).

Due to the inherent design of the exercises and equipment, much of the Pilates repertoire involves both isometric and isotonic contractions and emphasizes both the concentric and the eccentric phases of movement. Traditional weightlifting exercises tend to emphasize one or the other, most commonly the concentric phase. For example, when someone uses the biceps curl machine, the body and upper arm is supported by the structure of the machine, and one merely bends the elbow against resistance for a concentric biceps contraction. There is no emphasis on the eccentric phase as the machine assists with the lowering of the weight. This is not typical of real-life activities, and thus not a functional exercise. Contrast this with Pilates: due to the design of the equipment, muscles are worked both concentrically and eccentrically throughout the range of motion. Using springs and pulleys that create progressive resistance, the equipment helps in producing muscle contractions (eccentric, concentric, and isometric) that simulate functional muscle action.

The amount of muscle force produced varies by type of contraction. Eccentric contractions produce more force than either isometric or concentric contractions. Maximum eccentric strength is estimated to be between one and a half and two times maximum concentric strength (Bullock, Boyle, and Wang 2001). This is an important concept to keep in mind when selecting rehabilitation exercises. For a client whose tissues are still healing from a recent rotator cuff surgery, for example, the first phase of rehab would consist primarily of isometric and concentric exercises, so that the least amount of force is produced. As the shoulder heals and the muscles begin to regain their strength, we progress to eccentric exercises. The Pilates repertoire offers options for all of these types of contractions, making it easy to select the correct exercises for the patient's stage of healing.

5. Pilates Exercises Are Functional

The three previous fundamentals establish that Pilates exercises enhance both stability and mobility; include both open- and closed-chain exercises; and work the muscles statically and dynamically (emphasizing both concentric and eccentric phases). All of this leads us to reason 5: Pilates is a very functional type of exercise.

When functional movements such as walking or running are performed, a single muscle does not work in isolation. Such movements often involve multiple muscles—some working concentrically, some eccentrically, and some isometrically—in a highly coordinated manner to achieve the desired action. Many Pilates exercises simulate everyday activities, which makes them perfect for injury rehab and prevention. Looking again at the example of a biceps curl machine at the gym, the client is seated on a chair with the trunk completely supported and the arms resting on a platform. The motion is to bend the elbow against resistance, resulting in isolation of the biceps muscle and emphasis only on the concentric phase of the movement. How often in life do we need this type of strength? Not often unless we are arm wrestlers! More frequently we need to be able to perform such tasks as lifting our carry-on bag and placing it in the overhead compartment on a moving airplane. This takes not only dynamic (concentric and eccentric) upper extremity strength, but also scapular stabilization and core stabilization. An exercise such as the kneeling biceps on the reformer (p. 136) simulates this type of action.

The concept of functionality in rehab also means we must look at what the client needs and make our exercises task specific. Is your client a ballet dancer needing flexibility, a rugby player needing strength, a desk jockey needing postural exercises to reverse the effects of sitting all day, or an elderly woman who needs to be able to get up from a seated position? The huge repertoire of Pilates exercises provides endless options to allow us to make the exercises appropriate for all types of clients. If the exercise does not exist in the repertoire, we can design an appropriate exercise, using the equipment to either provide support or create additional challenge.

6. Pilates Places an Importance on Breathing Appropriately

As discussed during our review of the guiding principles in chapter 2, Pilates places an importance on breathing appropriately, which, among other things, enables us to activate key muscles. Lateral breathing is utilized to maintain

Breathing

- Oxygenates the blood and nourishes the body on a cellular level
- Expels toxins from the body
- Improves circulation
- Calms the mind and body
- Encourages concentration
- Provides a rhythm for movement

abdominal contraction throughout the breathing cycle. The specific breath pattern used (exhale during trunk flexion, inhale during trunk extension) enables us to emphasize activation of the key muscles in core stabilization. More details and the rationale for use of this breathing technique are addressed in chapter 2 (p. 16). There are many other benefits of deep, proper breathing that contribute to the injury rehabilitation process.

7. Pilates Is Adaptable for Many Different Patient Populations

Pilates is versatile and adaptable, and therefore appropriate for just about any patient or client who we may see. It offers a solution to those with restricted mobility and to elite athletes—from the 93-year-old woman with osteoporosis and a total hip arthroplasty to the professional athlete with an anterior cruciate ligament reconstruction. The Pilates system facilitates a positive movement experience no matter the patient's level, size, or limitations. The equipment allows us to select or create the appropriate exercises based on whether the patient's condition requires more support or increased challenge. It is as motivating for men as for women and it is safe for all ages when used correctly. What types of diagnoses can benefit from Pilates? Here is a sample list.

- Low back pain
- Neck pain
- Post–motor vehicle accident pain, stiffness, or instability
- Piriformis syndrome
- Patellofemoral pain syndrome
- Multiple sclerosis
- Amyotrophic lateral sclerosis
- Arthritis
- Sacroiliac joint dysfunction
- Total joint replacement (knee, hip, shoulder)
- Rotator cuff repair

- Arthroscopic surgery (knee, ankle, hip, shoulder)
- Sprained ankle
- Scoliosis
- Shoulder impingement
- Cerebrovascular accident
- Parkinson disease
- Poor flexibility
- Generalized weakness

8. Pilates Is a Mind–Body Form of Conditioning

In my experience, patients can reach far greater potential when mental conditioning is integrated into the motor learning and neuromuscular reeducation process. This is easily achieved by following the 10 guiding principles of Pilates presented in chapter 2. It is widely accepted that some version of these principles are what make Pilates a mind–body form of conditioning rather than only a physical process. As stated by physiotherapist, occupational therapist, and Pilates instructor trainer Wayne Seeto (2011), "Mindful movement and proper diaphragmatic breathing provide kinesthetic awareness and a stable base from which to move. The idea of focusing the mind on what the body is doing can afford profound benefits."

9. Pilates Equipment Is Safe and Easy to Use (With Proper Training)

The Pilates apparatus are safe and user friendly for those who are properly trained. However, they are potentially dangerous if not used correctly and with discretion. The springs are exposed, ropes and straps are hanging freely, and there are many adjustments on the apparatus. If incorrectly positioned, the patient could suffer injury, and if the teacher is spotting from the wrong position he or she risks injury as well. The equipment does not completely support the user; the user needs to support himself or herself. This of course makes the exercises very functional and part of why Pilates is so effective in athletic conditioning; yet it is also potentially dangerous for the inexperienced user. Proper training and experience with an apparatus is therefore crucial before working with patients. Specifics on safety when using the equipment will be covered in the next chapter.

10. Pilates Is a Wise Business Choice to Expand Your Wellness Services

Overhead costs for a sports medicine clinic or rehab center can be very expensive. Leasing a large enough space and purchasing the necessary equipment to provide quality wellness services can set business owners back thousands of dollars. Integrative use of Pilates, however, makes it much more affordable. Pilates equipment is not cheap, but hundreds of exercises can be done on one piece of equipment. Contrast this to a gym where there are multiple machines, each isolating a certain muscle group or area of the body. On the reformer, the most common Pilates apparatus, there are exercises for every area the body. Adding a Cadillac and a wunda chair makes the exercise options endless. Cadillacs and tower-style reformers can even be used as plinths for manual treatments. Because only one or a few apparatus are needed as opposed to 10 or 20 in a traditional gym setting, you can fit everything an injury rehab clinic or wellness center needs in a relatively small space. The result of these advantages is a significant reduction in square footage required and decreased overhead expenses.

In addition to integrating Pilates during physiotherapy treatment sessions, offering a postrehabilitation Pilates program offers many advantages for rehabilitation professionals. First, it allows business growth through a dual strategy of increasing the number of customers and expanding the services offered. Assuming you already have Pilates equipment, by hiring qualified instructors and developing a program, you can see significant revenue increases without incurring major increases in expenses. Stabilizing cash flow is an even greater benefit. When billing insurance companies for healthcare services, it can be difficult to manage cash flow as insurance payments tend to have a collection time from 30 to 60 days. Pilates clients pay for sessions in advance, which produces a predictable cash flow to help offset overhead and incremental expenses. Many patients who use Pilates in rehabilitation see the benefits of this form of exercise. They also enjoy it, so they're willing and even eager to pay out of pocket for these services, even after their insurance quits covering them (Wood 2004).

By offering postrehabilitation Pilates services, you increase awareness of your clinic and can bring more patients and clients to your core rehabilitation business. Customers also benefit from this union. Patients who go through rehab or prehab at your clinic and continue or return as Pilates clients after they cease to be patients have the reassurance that the Pilates instructor knows about their injuries because there has been communication with the PT, chiropractor, or athletic trainer. Furthermore, clients work out in a comfortable, safe, healing environment, instead of the traditional gym setting. They also have a fully qualified Pilates instructor trained and supervised by their rehab specialist. And finally, both client and instructor can consult with the PT, chiropractor, or athletic trainer whenever necessary (Wood 2004).

Importance of an Accurate Assessment

The primary purpose of rehabilitation is to produce a change in a patient's condition, both physically and mentally. It is our goal as rehab specialists to enable people to function optimally and pain free. In order to do this, we must first identify the patient's problems and limitations, both subjectively and objectively, and set appropriate goals based on these limitations. We can then plan and direct the actual treatment and specific exercises. Only when an accurate assessment is done can an effective treatment plan be prescribed.

In my physical therapy and wellness center, we do a comprehensive evaluation on the patient's initial visit, during which we take a thorough subjective history, assess posture and body mechanics, measure range of motion and strength, and perform any special tests applicable to the injury or pathology. During this session we also apply any necessary modalities (such as ice, heat, ultrasound, electrical stimulation, or tape) and perform any manual treatments that are appropriate for the patient's injury, such as joint or soft tissue mobilization. We teach the patient proper posture and body mechanics for their activities of daily living and issue a home exercise program. Often this program will include an introduction to some of the guiding principles (awareness, core engagement, breathing, etc.) and sometimes a couple of basic Pilates mat exercises, but very rarely do we begin integrating therapeutic exercise on the Pilates equipment on day one. The most important thing on this initial visit is performing an accurate assessment and creating a treatment plan to meet the patient's needs. Furthermore, it is important to continually reassess patients on subsequent visits to ensure the appropriateness of the exercises chosen and be able to modify as needed.

Even if two people have the exact same diagnosis, their presentation and specific issues can be very different. One status post–total knee replacement patient's most significant impairments could be weakness and swelling, while another's could be muscular tightness and impaired neuromuscular control. Adequate physiological and biomechanical knowledge and performance of an accurate assessment is needed to ensure that we are clear on any precautions or contraindications for the patient's pathology or injury. It is crucial that these are taken into account when prescribing the specific exercises. General precautions and contraindications will be covered in later chapters, but as an example, patients often come in with a diagnosis of low back pain. Based on this, we cannot prescribe appropriate exercises. A thorough subjective history and accurate objective assessment must be performed to determine the source of the back pain. If the pain is from a herniated disk, we would exclude trunk flexion exercises; but if it is due to spondylolisthesis, we would avoid trunk extension.

This rationale applies to athletes as well. Just because a person is an athlete does not mean we prescribe the same Pilates exercises for everyone. All sports have different mechanics, so to treat them all the same would be totally erroneous. Each sport has unique demands, so athletes need sport-specific conditioning and treatment. We need to identify the most vulnerable muscles to appropriately stretch and strengthen based on the athlete's sport. However, no matter what the sport is, research has shown that core muscles initiate and attenuate forces generated by the rotational movements of athletic performance (Donatelli 2009). Thus Pilates principles can help all athletes improve performance, reduce the risk of further injury, and maximize their training after effectively healing.

Pilates as a Tool

In physiotherapy, Pilates exercises are considered neuromuscular reeducation, therapeutic exercise, or therapeutic activity. The Pilates repertoire and apparatus are used as tools of the trade and adapted to the needs of each individual and his or her unique goals. The approach I use with patients is as follows: exercises are chosen and sequenced based on the specific needs of the patient while attempting to maintain the holistic approach of the work. Exercises are not changed to accommodate for movements the person may be accustomed to, but rather the individual adapts to corrections and positive movement patterns being taught. The goal then becomes achieving optimal posture, functional strength, and balance in the individual as well as rehabilitating the injury.

The first two chapters explained the guiding principles on which the Pilates method is based and presented scientific research advocating the use of Pilates in the injury rehab realm. In this chapter, I shared with you the fundamental reasons I think Pilates works so well for injury rehab and prevention. Some of these reasons are scientific, others practical, and others have more to do with the spiritual or mind–body connection. I have also shared with you how we integrate Pilates into our treatment plans at my physical therapy and wellness clinic. I hope that after reading this far, you'll agree that Pilates can be a valuable tool for rehab professionals to have in our toolboxes. In the following chapter, we will get into the actual methodology and apparatus used in Pilates.

4

Methodology and Apparatus Needed for an Effective Practice

The previous chapters laid the foundation for what Pilates is and why it is effective in injury rehab. This chapter will explain how we integrate Pilates into patient programs to help them heal from injuries and prevent new ones from occurring. Before getting into the actual exercises, it is essential to understand and learn to teach what I refer to as pre-Pilates methodology. There is a consensus among researchers, clinicians, and practitioners that the mind–body connection emphasized in Pilates is one explanation for its effectiveness. Remember the guiding principles: awareness, balance, breath, concentration, center, control, efficiency, flow, harmony, and precision. If we were to ignore these and dive right into the exercises we would simply be performing physical movements and thus missing out on some of the key benefits of Pilates. This would be an injustice to the method and to our patients.

Pre-Pilates Methodology

To fully understand and embody all of the guiding principles takes time. They cannot be taught in one session, one month, or even one year, but we can start with the basics: alignment (awareness and balance), Pilates breathing (breath), and finding and setting the core (concentration and center); and the rest will flow from there. It is important to keep in mind that there is a difference between teaching Pilates as simply a form of exercise and using it as a form of therapy. In this section, I will explain step by step how I use a combination of Pilates principles, scientific concepts, and therapeutic techniques to prepare patients for an effective practice.

Alignment

Before a client begins the actual Pilates exercises, it is important that he understands what good alignment is and how to achieve it. With good alignment, there is less stress on the spine and other joints, and muscular activity is more efficient. In Pilates and in lumbar spine rehabilitation, alignment begins with the neutral pelvis position. Neutral pelvis is a definable position that is the same for everyone. It refers to the position that results when the anterior superior iliac spine (ASIS) on each side of the pelvis and the pubic symphysis (PS) are on the same horizontal plane when supine (coronal plane when upright), and each ASIS is on the same transverse plane. An anterior tilt is when each ASIS is higher than (or anterior to when upright) the PS, resulting in an increased lumbar curve. A posterior tilt is when the PS is higher than (or anterior to when upright) the ASIS, resulting in a decreased lumbar curve (see figure 4.1).

When we are in the neutral pelvic position, the resulting spinal position is called neutral spine. This refers to the position of the spine in which all three natural curves are present; thus, it can be different for each person. It is well accepted in biomechanics that the position in which spinal curves are maintained is the most energy-efficient position for the body to stay upright against the forces of gravity and to withstand additional forces applied to the spine (Richardson, Jull, and Hodges 2004). When the spine is in a neutral position, the pelvis must also be in neutral. However, when the pelvis is in the neutral position, the spine is not. For example, when lying supine in neutral pelvic position, we will also be in neutral spine position; but once the head is lifted off the floor as in doing a sit-up, we can still be in neutral pelvis but not neutral spine as we are now in spinal flexion.

Neutral pelvis and neutral spine are reference points, the base from which we can compare and describe other positions. It is important that clients know how to find neutral, but it does not mean that all exercises should be done in this position. In fact, in certain circumstances it is actually better to deviate from neutral. For example, trying to maintain a neutral pelvis during exercises like the chest lift (p. 61) can place excess stress on the lower back. It is counterproductive to work with a neutral pelvis when the body cannot hold the position due to weakness, poor flexibility, muscle tightness, structural issues, or injury. A neutral pelvis may be the ideal, but with many clients it may be necessary, at

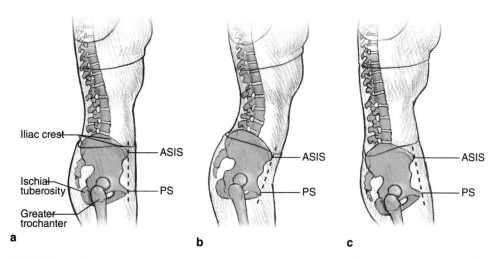

FIGURE 4.1 Pelvic alignment *(a)* neutral pelvis, *(b)* anterior tilt, and *(c)* posterior tilt.

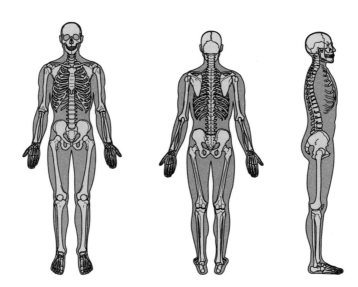

FIGURE 4.2 Standing alignment.

least in the beginning, to work in a posterior tilt in order to relax the lumbar extensor muscles and make it easier to access the abdominals.

As summarized by Rael Isacowitz in his workshop, "Pilates, Biomechanics and Reality" (2006), working in the neutral position is ideal for a few reasons: it is the most efficient position for generating force; it is the safest position to work in to protect the body against injury; it encourages correct and balanced recruitment of the core (local) muscles as well as the global muscles acting on the limbs; and it teaches and reinforces efficient posture and ideal alignment, thereby allowing functional and positive movement patterns. In addition, studies have shown that activation of TrA is more independent if there is no pelvis or spinal motion (Richardson et al. 2004; Urquhart et al. 2005). However, forcing a client to work in neutral spine before he is ready can result in ineffective abdominal work as well as exacerbate existing conditions such as neck tension or tight lower back muscles. The neutral position is therefore something we strive for in Pilates, but certain individuals may never achieve it.

Once the patient has been educated in neutral pelvis and neutral spine, it is important to look at other areas of the body. Ideally, optimal positioning and alignment of all these areas is achieved before beginning the exercises. Depending on body type, habitual patterns, and injuries or pathologies, each person will have deviations from the ideal. Figure 4.2 illustrates ideal alignment, and table 4.1 suggests some cues to help clients achieve it.

Pilates Breathing

As discussed in previous chapters, correct breathing is very important in Pilates and in rehabilitation to achieve optimal results.

TABLE 4.1   Cues to Achieve Ideal Alignment

Area	Ideal alignment	Cues to help achieve alignment
Head, cervical spine	Neutral, with slight upper cervical flexion so chin is not jutting forward Ears in line with shoulders	Slight chin nod Supine: slide back of head along mat, elongate the spine Upright: grow taller through the top of the head
Shoulder girdle	Shoulders in line with ears Shoulders open, not rounding forward Scapulae neutral—not elevated, depressed or protracted, retracted	Draw the shoulder blades down and back, as if placing them in back pockets Spread across the collarbones
Rib cage	Pulled in, not thrusting outward	Supine: press the back of your rib cage down into the mat or press the bra strap down into the mat Upright (against wall): press the back of the ribs into the wall
Thoracic and lumbar spine	Neutral	None needed; once neutral pelvis is achieved, neutral spine (natural curvature) is the result
Pelvis	Neutral	Supine: ASIS and PS on the same horizontal plane and ASIS on the same transverse plane Standing: ASIS and PS on the same coronal plane and ASIS on the same transverse plane
Knees	Knee joint directly below hip joint and directly above ankle joint Parallel—not knocking in (valgus) or bowing out (varus) Kneecap in line with space between second and third toes	Place a small ball between the knees or imagine a ball between the knees Imagine skiing down a hill
Feet	Parallel, hip distance apart Subtalar joint neutral—feet not rolled in (pronated) or rolled out (supinated)	Roll ankles in and out, then find the midpoint and hold Imagine skiing down a hill

In BASI Pilates, the basic breath pattern used is to exhale with spinal flexion and inhale with spinal extension. This provides a natural rhythm for movement, as well as assists in activating specific muscle groups.

To teach Pilates breathing, I generally start with the patient in a comfortable, supine position. I have the patient cross his or her arms over the belly and place his or her hands on the rib cage. Then I instruct the patient to take a deep breath in and feel the rib cage expand into his or her hands. On the exhale, the patient should feel the belly sink. For patients with neck pain, overuse of the anterior neck muscles during breathing (sternocleidomastoid [SCM] and scalene muscles) is often an issue. After teaching these patients lateral breathing in a supine position, I have them place one hand over the front of the neck while the other hand is on the belly. Although the belly and rib cage will still expand on inhalation and contract on exhalation, the patient should not feel any movement or tension in the anterior neck muscles.

Core Strength: Setting the Core

Once the client has learned proper alignment and breathing, it is time to learn to set the core. The importance of the deep stabilizing (core) muscles in injury rehabilitation has been well established both in the literature and in clinical practice. As discussed in previous chapters, the concept that all movement originates from the center or core is a common theme in Pilates, and much emphasis is placed on recruiting these core muscles for many, if not all of the exercises. This next section guides you through the methodology I use to teach patients to find and set the core (Withers and Bryant 2011).

Lower Core (Lumbo-Pelvic Core)

Patient position: supine, hook lying (knees bent, feet flat); pelvis in neutral position if attainable and not painful

Clinician position: at patient's side, with two fingers of one hand palpating approximately one inch (2.54 cm) in toward the belly button (medial) and one inch (2.54 cm) down from (inferior to) the ASIS, ideally between the rectus abdominis and obliques (see figure 4.3).

Instructions to the patient:

Method 1 (Lower Abdomen Cue)

Imagine a string attached to one hip bone (ASIS), running along the abdomen and attaching to the other hip bone. On an exhale, draw the belly down away from that string (the patient should be able to feel and the clinician should be able to see and feel the belly sink). The patient continues breathing normally for 10 seconds as the belly is held down away from the string (Withers and Bryant 2011).

Method 2 (Pelvic Floor Cue)

Engage the pelvic floor muscles by doing a Kegel. Maintain the Kegel while breathing for 10 seconds. If the patient does not understand what a Kegel is,

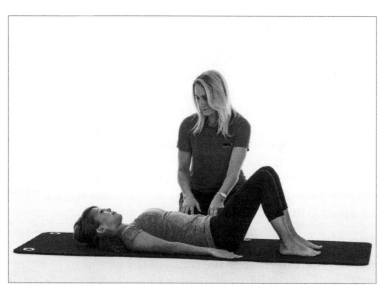

FIGURE 4.3 Setting the core.

other imagery to achieve activation of the pelvic floor muscles can be used (stop the flow of urine mid-stream, draw the testicles up, pull the bones of the pelvis together, etc.).

After the patient attempts both methods of engaging the core, decide which resulted in the most isolated activation of the TrA. As the TrA is the deepest layer of the abdominal muscles, it is difficult or in some cases impossible to truly see or feel it, so to know if it is functioning properly we need to feel and watch for other muscle activity. A strong bulging out or doming of the abdomen indicates activation of the more superficial abdominal muscles. An isolated contraction of the TrA is felt as a slow, gentle, minimally perceptible contraction. It should feel like the skin is tightening under your fingertips, not like a muscle is bulging out.

As discussed in chapter 3, we can postulate that with this activation of TrA, we are getting cocontraction of the other core muscles (multifidi, pelvic floor, and diaphragm). This abdominal drawing in maneuver, or imprinting, takes practice to get the correct firing patterns set, because these deep muscles are often inhibited by pain or inactivity. So once the patient understands what to do and how to do it, this becomes a daily practice. The goal is that when the patient is cued to center or set the core during the Pilates exercises, he or she will know exactly what to do.

Of course lying supine in neutral is not a functional position, but it is important to start in this pain-free, supported position to allow for the most isolated activity of the TrA (Richardson, Jull, and Hodges 2004), as well as muscular retraining and reorganization of the motor cortex (Tsao and Hodges 2007). Once the patient can perform the maneuver in the supine neutral position, we can move him or her to more functional and challenging positions such as sitting, standing, or lying on an unstable surface (foam roll, ball, or the moving carriage of the reformer).

Upper Core (Cervicothoracic Region)

For patients with neck pain or dysfunction, the ability to find and activate the upper core (discussed in chapter 3) is very important. Remembering the Pilates principles: good posture begins from the core, so first the patient must know how to correctly recruit the TrA and thus activate the lower core, as instructed previously in this chapter. However, the TrA runs only from the rib cage to the pubis, so when working specifically with cervical spine dysfunctions, we must also address the upper core. If this core is functioning properly, there is no reason for the muscles that are so often too tight (SCM, upper trapezius, and levator scapula) to have to overwork and cause neck tension. So, similar to how we teach patients to engage their lower core, we can teach them to engage their upper core.

Part I: Deep Neck Flexors

Similar to the TrA, we can neither see nor feel the DNFs, so to know if they are functioning properly we need to feel for other muscle activity. So in this exercise, just as we taught the patient to isolate the TrA without using the more superficial abdominal muscles; we teach the patient to isolate the DNFs without using the more superficial neck muscles (SCM and anterior scalenes [AS]).

Patient position: supine, hook lying. Cervical spine in neutral position, on a small pillow to reduce excessive lordosis and for comfort if necessary.

Clinician position: at the head of the patient, with a trigger-type grip of sub-occipitals (little fingers under occiput, middle fingers on the sides of the neck). This allows the clinician to guide the movement slightly, while at the same time feeling for muscle activation and watching for over-recruitment of the SCM and AS (see figure 4.4).

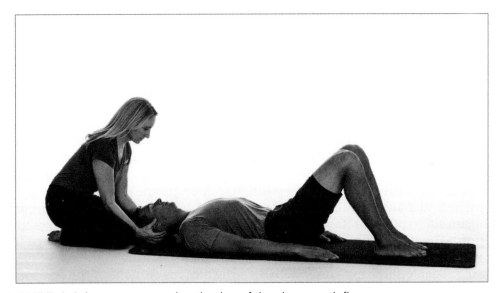

FIGURE 4.4 Assessment and activation of the deep neck flexors.

Instructions to the patient:

Step 1 *(activation of superficial anterior neck muscles)*: Place one hand on the front of your neck, over the anterior neck muscles. Lift your head off the mat, feeling the tightening and bulging of the SCM and AS. Gently lower the head back to the mat.

Note to clinician: the purpose of this step is for the patient to learn what muscles he or she should *not* feel when doing the chin nod.

Step 2 *(chin nod to activate DNF)*: Gently press the back of your head into the mat, bringing the chin into a gentle nod or tuck, while elongating through the back of the neck. Do all of this *without* feeling the bulge of the SCM and AS.

Note to clinician: As with the TrA, an isolated contraction of the DNF is felt as a slow, gentle, minimally perceptible contraction. It should feel like the skin is tightening under your fingertips, not like a muscle is bulging out.

Step 3 *(home exercise program to build strength and endurance of the DNF)*: Do a minimum of 10 chin nods with a 10-second hold daily. Once this becomes easy, progress to more functional positions such as sitting and standing.

The ability to do this simple exercise correctly indicates that the DNF are functioning properly and we can now move on to the next part of the upper core.

Part II: Lower Trapezius and Serratus Anterior

Patient position: prone propped up on elbows (sphinx pose), elbows slightly forward of the shoulders. Eyes looking down at the floor so the head is slightly down, and the cervical spine is in a neutral position to slight flexion.

Clinician position: sitting to the side of the patient, with the thumb and first finger of one hand at inferior angles of the patient's scapulae, thumb and first finger of the other hand on the patient's sternum (optional) (see figure 4.5).

Instructions to the patient

Step 1: Set the lower core.

Step 2: Activate the DNF by performing a chin nod.

Step 3: Activate the lower trapezius by drawing the shoulder blades down and back, as if placing them in the opposite back pocket. Visualize spreading wide across the collar bones. Be sure to do this *without* tensing the anterior neck muscles, upper trapezius, or levator scapulae.

Step 4: To activate the serratus anterior, press down into the elbows and float the breast bone away from the floor (or from the clinician's hand if palpating breastbone) while maintaining the chin nod and shoulder blade position. Do not lift the head or tense the neck muscles.

Note to clinician: Sometimes the breast bone cue causes people to round their shoulders and overuse the pecs. If this happens, remove your fingers from the patient's sternum and try instead cueing the patient to push the elbows down into the mat as the back of the rib cage elevates.

This section has explained what the client needs to learn and practice before beginning a Pilates program. Whether you use the exact methodology I've

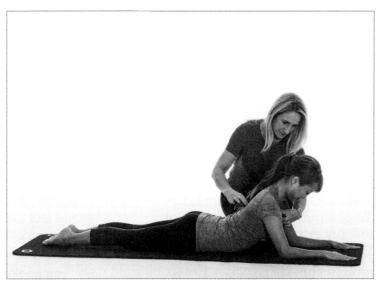

FIGURE 4.5 Activation of the lower trapezius and serratus anterior.

guided you through or some of your own, the important thing is that the client learns these pre-Pilates basics—alignment, breathing, and finding and setting the core(s)—before beginning the actual exercises. Also remember that there is a difference between teaching Pilates as simply a form of exercise and using it as a form of therapy. If the exercises are not used in conjunction with the therapeutic concepts and techniques discussed, they could aggravate injuries.

Now that we have covered the what, why, and how of integrating Pilates into therapeutic treatments, we are almost ready to learn the actual exercises. But first, it is important to be introduced to the equipment and to learn how to use it safely.

Apparatus

Today there are many different pieces of Pilates apparatus—some invented by Joseph Pilates himself, and some more recent innovations. In addition to the larger equipment, there are many accessories now commonly used in Pilates studios (balls, foam rolls, etc.). All of them are wonderful to have, but in this section I am only covering the larger Pilates apparatus used in part II of this book. I feel that these are the most appropriate in an injury rehab and prevention or therapeutic setting.

Spring Tension

Pilates equipment is unique in its use of springs, rather than weights as in traditional gym equipment. The type of resistance provided by springs is termed *progressive resistance*. The amount of resistance is determined by the thickness or strength of the spring and the amount of stretch or tension on it. When lifting weights, the weight (resistance) remains constant throughout the range of motion, but due to the principle of mechanical advantage or disadvantage, the muscle effort required changes according to the varying angles of the joint(s). With spring resistance, however, the resistance increases as the spring is further tensioned, resulting in the muscle being challenged throughout the full range. Both types of resistance, though different, are effective and important in muscular development.

One advantage of springs over weights is that they can be more easily adapted to simulate many other activities and are therefore more functional (Isacowitz 2005). For injury rehabilitation, spring resistance is safer because at the beginning phase of a repetition, the resistance can be released, relieving any compression on the joint or pressure on the muscle.

One of the difficulties of working with springs, however, is that the spring settings vary from one piece of equipment to another, and even the same piece of equipment will vary from manufacturer to manufacturer. Unfortunately, there is no universal standard. For this reason, instead of giving an exact spring setting for each exercise, I use a resistance range, which translates to a limited number of spring setting positions.

It is also important to realize that the terms heavy or light are relative and will vary by the exercise: two springs on the reformer is light for footwork but heavy for arm work. Appropriate spring tension for any given exercise will vary from person to person depending on height, weight, body proportions, skill level, and injury or pathology. For example, arms supine series on the reformer (p. 97) might require two to three springs for a 200-pound male rugby player, but half to one spring for a 110-pound female recovering from rotator cuff surgery. When using the Pilates method with your patients, it is crucial that you are intricately familiar with the resistance settings on each piece of equipment so that you can determine the correct spring resistance for every person and every exercise.

Mat

Though perhaps not truly an apparatus, the mat work is the foundation of the Pilates system, so it deserves mention here. Mat exercises are always the first I teach my patients—not because they are the easiest, but because they are the root of all other exercises in the Pilates repertoire. If one is not familiar with the mat work, one lacks the foundation necessary to develop a powerful Pilates practice. From a practical standpoint, mat exercises can be practiced anywhere, anytime. Most people do not have a reformer or other Pilates equipment in their homes, so the mat exercises serve as their home exercise program. I find that if the patient practices some fundamental mat exercises between sessions, he or she is able to internalize the principles and movements of Pilates much faster. This of course allows us to progress safely to the equipment.

Reformer

The most commonly recognized and popular apparatus used in Pilates is the reformer (see figure 4.6). Though most Pilates studios and Pilates-based rehab centers have the full suite of equipment, if you can only afford one piece, I

Genius of the Equipment

- Allows for different orientations to gravity (prone → supine → seated → kneeling → standing)
- Provides both stable and moving surface options
- Extreme adjustability
- Creates both support and resistance
- Teaches proprioception and balance in addition to strength and flexibility

recommend the reformer. Of all the Pilates equipment, the reformer offers the most variety of movements, and it accommodates movement throughout the full range of motion as adjustments can be made according to patient size and limitations. Exercises done on the reformer range from fundamental to extremely advanced and include all positions: supine, prone, sitting, kneeling, and standing. The reformer even allows cardio exercise and plyometrics with use of the jump board attachment. The possibilities are vast on the reformer, limited only by our understanding of the equipment and of course our creativity.

From a rehab standpoint, I prefer working on the reformer, especially in the initial stages of rehab or prehab, because it provides a wonderful viewpoint for both the client and the instructor from which to observe alignment and muscular patterning. It also allows a patient to be positioned in such a way as to help remove gravity from the equation, allowing for earlier progressive load bearing. For example, with an exercise such as footwork on the reformer (p. 88), natural upright alignment of the body is reinforced, and we can begin functional exercises such as squatting without worrying about too much compression on the patient's joints. This is invaluable for patients who have difficulty standing or walking due to arthritic joints, surgical weight-bearing restrictions, generalized weakness, or balance issues. We can still work on upright posture and alignment, as well as lower extremity strength, without stressing the joints or putting the patient at risk of falling. This allows for exact functional patterns and muscle memory to be retrained and so that when the patient is ready to bear weight into a squat or lunge, the motion has already been learned.

Parts of the Reformer (see figure 4.6)

Frame: The rigid structure that surrounds the apparatus. Made of either wood or aluminum, depending on manufacturer and model. Available in different heights.

Carriage: The moving platform.

Spring bar: The bar to which the springs attach. Generally two or three settings available.

Closer to the carriage = less spring tension

Closer to the frame = more spring tension

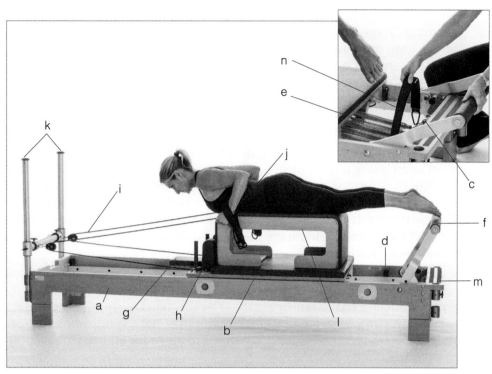

FIGURE 4.6 Reformer: *(a)* frame; *(b)* carriage; *(c)* spring bar; *(d)* stoppers; *(e)* springs; *(f)* foot bar; *(g)* head rest; *(h)* shoulder rests; *(i)* ropes; *(j)* loops and handles; *(k)* pulley risers; *(l)* box; *(m)* base; *(n)* foot strap.

Stoppers: Removable pegs that insert into holes on the tracks of the frame. Placing the stoppers in the holes closest to the foot bar allows for the most range of motion of the carriage, while placing the stoppers in the holes farthest from the foot bar allows for the least range of motion of the carriage.

Springs: The springs provide resistance as discussed previously. Spring tension on the reformer is as follows:

Extra light = half spring (25 to 50 percent)

Light = one to one and a half springs

Medium = two to three springs

Heavy = three and a half to four springs

Extra heavy = four and a half to five springs

Some manufacturers color code individual springs to designate the resistance:

Yellow = quarter or extra light

Blue = half or light

Red = one or medium

Green = one and a half, or heavy

Foot bar: A foot bar generally has three or four different settings, depending on manufacturer and model. It can be adjusted to accommodate the size of the patient or range of motion restrictions or goal of the exercise. For example, the bar can be placed in the lowest position when working with a taller person or a post-op total hip replacement patient to keep him or her in <90 degrees of hip flexion. Conversely, the bar can be placed in the highest position for a person with shorter legs or when the goal is to increase active flexion range of motion for a post-op total knee replacement patient.

Headrest: A headrest generally has three settings—up, neutral, or low. For most exercises it is kept in neutral, but it can be adjusted to accommodate posture or injury or pathology. For example, up is more comfortable for a patient with severe kyphosis, but down is better for someone with cervical disk pathology. If there are no contraindications, I like to use the up position for most exercises to encourage the neuromuscular connection often lacking in patients with injuries.

Shoulder rests: Classically immovable, certain manufacturers now make these adjustable in up to six positions. This allows wider and narrower spacing for larger or smaller framed individuals, as well as relief of shoulder compression for certain pathologies (e.g., shoulder impingement syndrome). Adjustable shoulder rests can also be easily removed to allow for an even greater variety of exercises.

Ropes: In more classical style reformers, these are leather straps. They can be adjusted shorter or longer.

Loops and handles: There are different varieties of grips available—handles, loops, fuzzy loops (covered with sheepskin), and even straps that go around the wrists for patients who are unable to grip.

Pulley risers: These are generally left in the center, but they can be adjusted to change the height and thus line of pull on the ropes to accommodate specific exercises. BASI Systems' enhanced pulley system allows fine tuning control of pulley angles to allow for isolation of desired muscle groups.

Box: A box is referred to as a long box when placed with the long side of the box parallel with the long axis of the reformer and a short box when placed with the short side of the box perpendicular with the long axis of the reformer. It is generally placed in front of the shoulder rests.

Base: The small platform at the foot bar end of the reformer. One of the main uses of this is for standing exercises. However, I recommend an oversized standing platform for increased exercise repertoire and safety.

Foot strap: A strap that hangs under the spring bar which can be placed over the feet to stabilize the body for certain exercises.

Jump board: The detachable board that fits into the foot bar end or base of the reformer. It allows for the jumping series of exercises (plyometrics) and is also useful for patients who need more surface area and stability than is provided by the foot bar (e.g., those with an ankle sprain or neurological condition such as multiple sclerosis or Parkinson disease). To see the jump board in use, refer to pages 162-164 in chapter 6.

Cadillac

The Cadillac is the largest and most expensive Pilates apparatus, and as such, it is not as commonly used in Pilates-based rehabilitation centers. But if you have the resources, I highly recommend it. The height and width make it very user friendly and safe for elderly or frail clients, and those with range-of-motion restrictions. It is also very stable, which is great for people who are uncomfortable with the moving platform of the reformer. It can be used as a plinth for joint and soft-tissue mobilization, proprioceptive neuromuscular facilitation (PNF), or manual stretching. A huge variety of exercises is possible—from gentle, spring-assisted roll-ups to advanced acrobatics. Due to its design, it challenges the body in multiple planes of motion. As with the reformer and chair, exercises can be done in prone, supine, side lying, sitting, kneeling, and standing positions on the apparatus. There are also some wonderful functional exercises that are done standing on the floor next to the Cadillac and using its springs or bars for resistance or support. The top bars even allow for hanging upside down, and the speed rails make it possible to provide traction when needed (see figure 4.7).

Parts of the Cadillac (see figure 4.7)

Frame or poles: Vertical poles and horizontal poles run along the sides and top of the apparatus. The push-through bar is attached on one side of the side poles, and the crossbar is on the other. Foot straps and a crossbar from which the trapeze hangs is on the top rails, which allows for some wonderful hanging and traction type exercises.

Sliding crossbars (speed rails): Crossbars glide left and right on the top poles or up and down on the upright poles. Both have eyelets from which to hang springs to provide resistance or support for exercises. The crossbar on the upright poles works well as an assist to enhance stability and positioning for certain exercises and stretches.

Springs: The springs provide resistance for the exercises. Most Cadillacs have multiple springs and multiple attachments. Cadillac springs come in long (for leg springs) and short (for arm springs) and in varying resistance.

Arm springs: very light (yellow), light (blue), medium (red), and heavy (green)

Leg springs: very light (yellow) and medium or heavy (purple)

Push-through bar (PTB): This is a very strong swinging bar that is able to carry a lot of weight, as there are exercises in which the weight of the whole body is reliant on the PTB. Springs can be loaded from the top (generally providing assistance) or the bottom (providing resistance). The bar swings so that it can be used on the inside or the outside of the apparatus, allowing for a huge

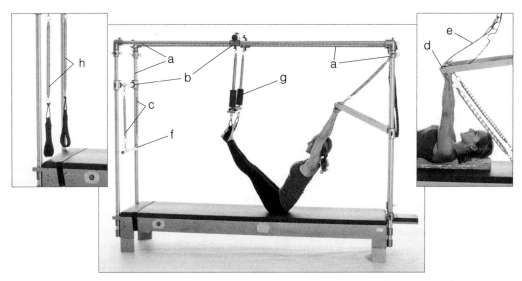

FIGURE 4.7 Cadillac: *(a)* frame or poles; *(b)* sliding crossbars (speed rails); *(c)* springs; *(d)* push-through bar (PTB); *(e)* safety strap; *(f)* roll-up bar; *(g)* trapeze bar or swing; *(h)* leg springs.

variety of exercises.

Safety strap: A safety strap must be used for certain positions and exercises so that the spring-loaded bar does not pop up and hit the client or instructor. It can also be used to keep the PTB securely out of the way when not in use.

Roll-up bar: This is a wooden bar on springs that hooks on to the eyelets of the crossbar or poles, providing resistance or in some cases support.

Trapeze bar or swing: A trapeze bar is used for hanging exercises and for support of the legs in exercises such as breathing with push-through bar (p. 167).

Note: Space-and cost-saving options include a reformer with a tower and a reformer-Cadillac combo, which are available from some manufacturers. These function as both a reformer and a Cadillac in one piece of convertible equipment. Most, but not all Cadillac exercises can be done on the reformer with the tower, whereas the combo reformer converts to a full Cadillac with all of the trapeze functionality.

Wunda Chair

The Pilates *wunda* (German for *wonder*) chair is basically a box-shaped chair with one side that can be pressed down against the resistance of springs. The original chair had a large, single pedal, but this has evolved into a split-pedal version. I recommend this version for rehab, because the pedal portion is divided into two independent parts, which allows for unilateral and reciprocal work; this is great for patients with one side that is weaker than the other due to injury or surgery, as well as for patients with a structural imbalance such as scoliosis. Exercises can be done on the chair in supine, prone, sitting, kneeling, and standing positions as well as from the floor adjacent to the front, back, or sides of the chair. The wunda chair is a key piece of equipment to have in a Pilates-based rehab center, because it is versatile, lightweight, and relatively inexpensive; doesn't take up too much space; and allows for many weight-bearing functional exercises. Though the chair lends itself to many great core and upper extremity exercises, I use it most for rehab and prehab of patients with hip and knee injuries or balance issues. It is a great tool for progressing weight-bearing status, from the supine zero-gravity position on the reformer to unsupported sitting and eventually standing exercises on the chair (see figure 4.8).

Parts of the Wunda Chair (see figure 4.8)

Seat: The width and depth of the seat varies by manufacturer and model. A larger seat is more user friendly and allows for more exercise options.

Pedals or foot bar: The original wunda chair had a single pedal, but most manufacturers now have split pedals available, which allows for unilateral work and reciprocal movement of the extremities.

Springs: The springs provide resistance for the exercises. Most chairs have a

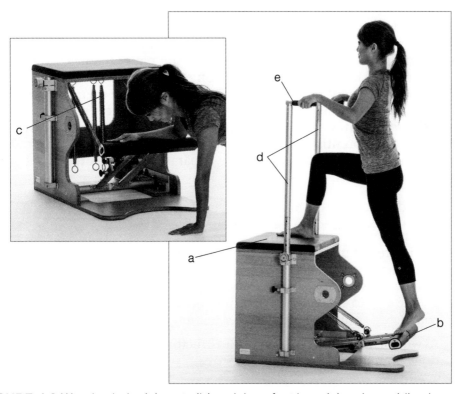

FIGURE 4.8 Wunda chair: *(a)* seat; *(b)* pedals or foot bar; *(c)* springs; *(d)* poles; *(e)* handles.

total of four springs—two light and two heavy—one of each on each pedal. There are many differences among manufacturers in the resistance adjustment system, and most of them are a bit cumbersome and can be somewhat difficult to standardize. The BASI Systems' wunda chair has an innovative pedal design that extends mobility and offers smoother transitions and adjustability of spring tension.

Spring settings on the chair:

> Lightest = one light spring (usually white) at the lowest position on one pedal

> Heaviest = two heavy springs (usually black) at the highest position on each pedal

Poles or handles: The poles are easily removable as they are necessary for some exercises or clients, but actually hinder others. They are also adjustable for height, and in some models angle.

Safety

In addition to following all the general protocols for exercise, Pilates requires particular attention to safety from both the instructor and the client due to the unique apparatus used. Pilates is often thought of as being safe and user friendly, but in reality, the equipment is potentially dangerous, and the method itself can be dangerous if not used correctly and with discretion. The springs are exposed, ropes and straps are hanging freely, and there are many adjustments on each apparatus. If incorrectly positioned, the patient could suffer injury, and if the teacher is spotting from the wrong position the teacher risks injury as well. The equipment does not completely support the user; the user needs to support him- or herself. This of course makes the exercises very functional and part of why Pilates is so effective in rehabilitation and athletic conditioning; yet it is also potentially dangerous for the inexperienced. Proper training in the method and experience with the apparatus is therefore crucial before working with patients.

Safety Guidelines

Adapted from the BASI Pilates Teacher Training Manual, Isacowitz, 2008.

- The instructor must be familiar with each exercise down to the finest detail, including any possible precautions or contraindications. This book is merely a guide to using Pilates for specific purposes. To truly embody the method and be able to successfully teach it to others, I feel strongly that one must complete a comprehensive teacher training course.

- As with any exercise program, the instructor must know the client's restrictions, limitations and medical history.

- Both instructor and student must be aware of the inherent dangers of all of the Pilates apparatus being used—springs, bars, straps, etc.

- Instructors should always assist clients when getting on and off the equipment, and when donning or doffing the straps (particularly the leg straps).

- We instructors must protect our own bodies by cueing and assisting from a safe position, yet one from which we are still able to support the weight of the client if necessary. It takes a lot of practice on the equipment to master this.

- Never change any springs when they are on tension.

- Only allow the patient to change position when there is no tension on the springs.

- The apparatus should be serviced regularly, including frequent checks on the condition of the springs. Springs should be replaced at the first sign of deterioration.

Specific Safety Points on the Reformer

- Never leave the reformer without any springs attached, whether there is a client on it or not. An unloaded reformer means the carriage will slide, which can be dangerous if someone does not realize this and attempts to sit down on the apparatus.

- Only change springs when the carriage is all the way in closest to the foot bar.

- Use an oversized standing platform for all standing exercises.

- Place the headrest in the down position during all exercises that place pressure on the cervical spine.

- Always move slowly and with consistent tension in the ropes. Quick, jerky movements cause the ropes to go slack, making some exercises ineffective and others a recipe for disaster.

Specific Safety Points on the Cadillac

- Always attach the safety strap when the springs are bottom loaded on the Cadillac. This prevents the bar from being pulled forcefully by the springs and striking the student or instructor.

- Use caution when the PTB is top loaded on the Cadillac. If a spring-loaded bar is suddenly released, it pops up very quickly and can strike the instructor or client.

Now that we have covered how to teach clients what they need to know before beginning a Pilates program, and you are familiar with the apparatus used, we can delve into the actual physical movements. Please note that there are hundreds of exercises from the classical repertoire alone, as well as hundreds of modifications and new creations, resulting in thousands of exercises that may be considered Pilates. The exercises in this book were selected due to both their simplicity for the novice practitioner and their role in injury rehab.

PART II

EXERCISES

5

Mat Exercises

Each exercise in this chapter and in the following chapters describes the physical Pilates movements with detailed instruction, primary muscles involved, objectives, indications, precautions or contraindications, variations and progressions as appropriate, and technique tips for correct execution. The exercise instructions are written in a voice such that a professional can instruct a client, or that the directions can be followed by the practitioner himself or herself. I recommend that anyone who does not have experience with Pilates works with a certified instructor to practice the exercises, both in the role of the client and of the teacher, before applying them in a rehabilitation practice. This is essential in being able to provide a safe and effective exercise program.

As the mat work is the foundation of the Pilates system, it is important to start here. After teaching the pre-Pilates methodology as described in chapter 4, a mat exercise such as the pelvic curl (p. 57), is usually one of the first exercises I teach to patients. This seemingly simple exercise emphasizes correct recruitment of the core, articulation of the spine, mobilization of the pelvic region, and coordination of breath pattern with movement. It is very difficult for people, especially when they are in pain or lack body awareness to focus on all of that while on a large, strange-looking apparatus that moves! It is much better to learn the correct execution of the exercise on solid ground where one feels relaxed and supported. Once the patient is comfortable with the mat version of the exercise, we can then perform the same exercise on the equipment, adding elements of challenge as appropriate (e.g., bottom lift with extension on the reformer, p. 95, pelvic curl with roll-up bar on the Cadillac, p. 165, and pelvic curl on the wunda chair, p. 196).

I want to emphasize, though, that mat work is definitely *not* the easiest of the Pilates work. In fact, it can be the most difficult. In many cases, the equipment helps to support the user or provides stabilization, which makes the exercise more approachable. In the mat work, the user must support himself or herself, and this can take much more experience and strength to safely achieve. Despite how difficult it can be, often the mat work is a great place for people to get started in Pilates. It is affordable, approachable, and easy to integrate into different settings. It can be used in a variety of ways: as a group class to promote strength and endurance in a flowing sequence, as a warm-up for a Pilates equipment session or other athletic activity, as a 5- to 10-minute personal daily conditioning program, as a home exercise program for injury rehabilitation, or for general body awareness and neuromuscular reeducation.

PELVIC CURL

Primary Muscles Involved

Abdominals, hamstrings, and gluteus maximus

Objectives

Mobilization of the spine and pelvic region, spinal articulation, hamstring control, pelvic lumbar stabilization, and recruitment and cocontraction of the core muscles

Indications

This is usually one of the first exercises I teach to patients, as it is relatively simple yet emphasizes the correct recruitment of the core, articulation of the spine, mobilization of the pelvic region, and coordination of the breath pattern with movement. Though challenging to execute correctly, even an attempt is beneficial for patients learning the concepts of neutral spine position and core control. It is great for those with general stiffness or arthritis of the spine, a weak or inhibited core, or tightness of back extensors or hip flexors.

Precautions or Contraindications

Acute lumbar disk pathology and osteoporosis

Instructions

Lie supine with the knees bent, legs parallel approximately hip distance apart, arms relaxed at the sides with palms down, and the pelvis in a neutral position (see photo *a*). Inhale to prepare, exhale to set the core, and begin to curl the pelvis and spine off the mat, one vertebra at a time. Inhale and hold at the top; the pelvis should be at maximum posterior tilt and a stretch should be felt in the hip flexors (see photo *b*). Exhale as the spine is lowered, starting at the thoracic vertebra and rolling down one vertebra at a time until the tailbone touches the mat.

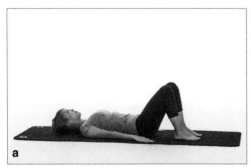
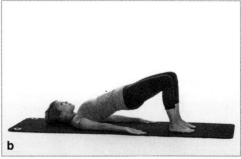

Variations

1. For disk pathologies, omit the deep lumbar flexion and maintain the spine and pelvis in neutral as it is lifted.
2. Place a ball between the knees to promote more adductor engagement and reach the arms overhead as the pelvis lifts to elicit more upper spine control (see photo *c*).

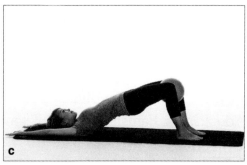

Progression

1. Feet placed on a foam roll (see photo *d*)
2. Bottom lift on reformer (p. 94)
3. Pelvic curl with roll-up bar on Cadillac (p. 165)
4. Pelvic curl on wunda chair (p. 196)

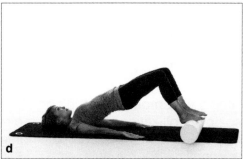

Technique Tips

1. Keep the neck and shoulders relaxed.
2. Maximize lumbar flexion as the spine lifts off the mat by pulling the pubic bone toward the chin (posteriorly tilting the pelvis).
3. Visualize the lowering of the spine like a Slinky spring toy going down steps, deliberately placing one vertebra at a time. This will help to achieve maximum articulation and spinal mobility.

SINGLE-LEG LIFTS

Primary Muscles Involved

Abdominals and hip flexors

Objectives

Lumbo-pelvic stabilization, hip joint dissociation, and abdominal and hip flexor control

Indications

Because this exercise is done in a neutral position of the spine, it allows for strengthening of the core muscles without going into often contraindicated positions of trunk flexion or extension. This is a great exercise for patients lacking pelvic stability or core awareness. Lifting one leg (open chain) in the sagittal plane as the other is on the mat (closed chain) begins to challenge the core in a functional way, similar to walking.

Precautions or Contraindications

Iliopsoas bursitis, severe hip flexor tightness, or acute hip flexor injury

Instructions

Lie supine with bent knees, parallel legs, relaxed arms at the sides with palms down, and neutral pelvic position (see photo a). Exhale as one leg is lifted to the tabletop position (90 degrees of hip and knee flexion) (see photo b). Inhale and return to the starting position by lowering the leg to the mat. Repeat with the same leg 5 to 10 times or alternate sides to increase pelvic stability challenge and to make it more functional.

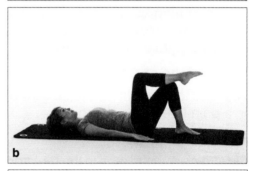

Progression

1. Leg changes: Lift one leg as the other leg lowers.
2. Perform the exercise lying on a half or full foam roll (see photo c).

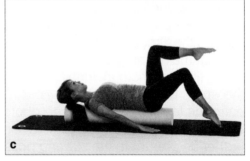

Technique Tips

1. Maintain a neutral pelvis throughout the exercise, especially avoiding hyperlordosis as the leg lowers.
2. Keep the neck and shoulders relaxed.
3. Keep the angle of the knee joint at 90 degrees throughout.
4. Imagine floating the legs up and down rather than lifting.

SUPINE SPINE TWIST

Primary Muscles Involved

Abdominals (emphasis on obliques)

Objectives

Spinal rotation, abdominal control with oblique emphasis, and pelvic lumbar stabilization

Indications

This is a great exercise for patients lacking spinal mobility (e.g., osteoarthritis or people with general stiffness). It helps to develop abdominal control, especially of the obliques, and challenges lumbo-pelvic stability in the transverse plane. This exercise is performed in a neutral position, thus allowing for strengthening of the core muscles without going into often contraindicated positions of trunk flexion or extension.

Precautions or Contraindications

None as long as the exercise is kept in a pain-free range of motion

Instruction

Lie supine with the legs in the tabletop position, ankles in line with the knees, arms in a *T* position with palms facing up, and the lumbar spine pressing into the mat maintaining a slight posterior pelvic tilt (see photo *a*). Inhale to rotate the spine and move the pelvis, lowering the legs to one side (see photo *b*). Exhale to draw the abdominals in farther and return to the starting position. Alternate sides.

Variations

1. Place both feet on the floor to make the exercise easier for those with lower back pain, hip flexor tightness, or lack of abdominal control.
2. Support the legs and feet on a large exercise ball (see photo *c*).

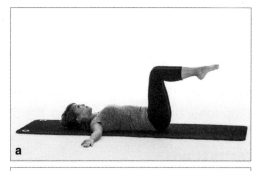

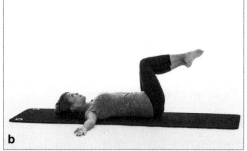

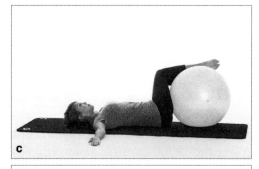

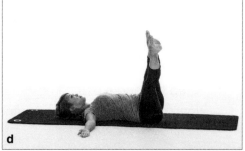

Progression

Begin as in photo *a*, but extend both legs when in the rotated position and keep the legs extended as you return to the starting position (see photo *d*). Bend the knees back to the tabletop position and repeat on the opposite side.

Technique Tips

1. The amount of rotation is dictated by flexibility and abdominal control. It is important to maintain contact of the lower back on the mat, thus avoiding hyperlordosis.
2. Keep the shoulders relaxed with the scapulae on the mat.
3. Keep the knees squeezed together and the feet in line with each other.
4. Think of focusing the movement in the waist area, initiating with the transversus abdominis (TrA) followed by the obliques.
5. The pelvis, knees, and feet should move as one unit. Do not let them glide back and forth over each other.

CHEST LIFT

Primary Muscles Involved

Abdominals

Objectives

Abdominal strength and lumbo-pelvic stability

Indications

Though this exercise resembles the crunch or sit-up, the emphasis is on engagement of the TrA, maintaining cocontraction of the core muscles throughout the movement, and pelvic stability. Momentum, pulling or tension in the neck area, and overuse of the hip flexors are all eliminated.

Precautions or Contraindications

Disk pathology, osteoporosis, and acute neck pain

Instruction

Lie supine in a neutral pelvic position (if tolerated and appropriate) with bent knees, legs parallel approximately hip-width apart, fingers interlaced with the hands cradling the head at the base of the neck (see photo *a*). On an inhale set the core muscles, then exhale to lift the head and chest as one unit. Continue lifting the upper spine until the inferior angles of the scapulae are off the mat (see photo *b*). Inhale, drawing the abdominals in even deeper as the height

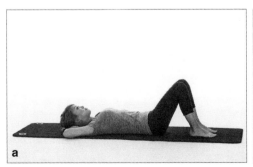
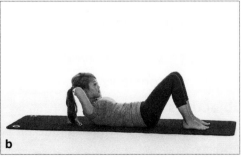

of the trunk is maintained. Exhale to lower the head and chest back to the starting position without releasing the abdominals.

Variations

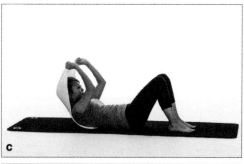

1. Have patients with tight back extensors or weak abdominals perform the exercise in a slight posterior tilt.

2. Have patients with neck pain or upper core weakness perform the exercise with a towel supporting the upper back and head (see photo *c*).

3. Patients with flexion restrictions (disk pathology, osteoporosis) should perform over the spine corrector or a physio ball (see photo *d*).

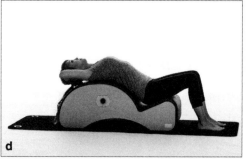

Progression

Chest lift with rotation (p. 62), hundred prep on the reformer (p. 102)

Technique Tips

1. Maintain a neutral position throughout the exercise, keeping the hip flexors relaxed and avoiding a posterior tilt of the pelvis (unless doing variation 1).

2. Keep the adductors engaged. Squeezing a small ball or block between the knees is useful if this is an issue.

3. Avoid pulling on the neck or leading with the chin. Engaging the upper core as described in chapter 4 (p. 42) is useful if this is an issue.

4. Keep the head aligned with the spine and imagine lengthening through the top of the head (elongating the spine).

5. Keep the gaze between the knees when lifted, rather than looking up to the ceiling.

CHEST LIFT WITH ROTATION

Primary Muscles Involved

Abdominals (primarily obliques)

Objectives

Abdominal strength with oblique emphasis, lumbo-pelvic stability, and spinal mobility

Indications

This exercise offers all the benefits of the chest lift, and adding spinal rotation challenges the abdominals even further due to the increased load placed on the obliques in a bilateral pattern. It is a very functional exercise especially for athletes because it develops pelvic stability coupled with spinal rotation, which is so important in everyday activities as well as most sports.

Precautions or Contraindications

Disk pathology, osteoporosis, and acute neck pain

Instructions

In the up position of the chest lift (see photo *a*) exhale as the upper girdle is rotated to one side (see photo *b*). Inhale, return to the starting position, and then exhale as the upper girdle is rotated to the opposite side (see photo *c*). Inhale and return to the starting position. Maintain the height of the upper girdle throughout the exercise.

Variations

1. For patients with tight back extensors or weak abdominals, allow the exercise to be performed in a slight posterior tilt.
2. If trunk flexion is contraindicated, perform over a BOSU balance trainer, physio ball, or core arc or spine corrector (see photo *d*) and keep the range of motion between extension and neutral.

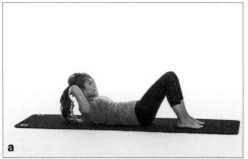
a

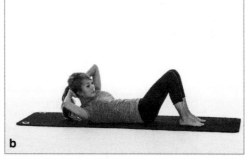
b

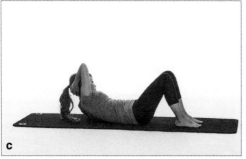
c

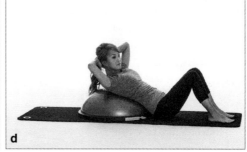
d

Technique Tips

1. Rotate through the waist, avoiding lateral flexion.
2. Maintain the stability of the pelvis.
3. Move the head, arms, shoulder girdle, and upper trunk as one unit.
4. Avoid pulling on the neck or leading with the chin. Engaging the upper core, as described in chapter 4 (p. 42), is useful if this is an issue.
5. Keep the distance between the elbows wide.

PRE-HUNDRED PREP (LEVELS 1, 2, 3)

Primary Muscles Involved

Abdominals (emphasis on TrA)

Objectives

Abdominal strength, trunk stabilization, and lumbo-pelvic control

Indications

A signature exercise of classical Pilates, the hundred, and even its prep exercise, are both very difficult and contraindicated for many pathologies. These modified versions are very useful for developing the ability to sustain cocontraction of the core muscles during breathing and arm movement but with the elimination of trunk flexion, making them appropriate for disk pathologies and osteoporosis. Progressing through these exercise levels challenges abdominal control and lumbo-pelvic stability incrementally via increasing the amount of open-chain sagittal plane movement (and thus load) of the arms and legs.

Precautions or Contraindications

Level 3 only: Contraindications include acute disk pathology, acute sacroiliac joint dysfunction or pain, and acute low back pain. Patients should be able to perform all three levels of pre-hundred prep correctly and without pain before moving on to the hundred prep.

Instruction

Level 1 (No Load on Lumbar Spine)

Lie supine with the knees bent, feet on the mat parallel to each other approximately hip distance apart, with the arms straight at the sides just hovering off the mat with palms down, and the pelvis in a neutral position (if tolerated and appropriate). Set the core and then pump the arms up and down in a small movement, exhaling for five pumps and inhaling for five pumps. Repeat up to 10 cycles (see photo *a*).

Level 2 (Partial Load on Lumbar Spine)

The starting position is the same as for level 1. Exhale to lift one leg to the tabletop position, then inhale and hold the position (see photo *b*). Pump the arms up and down for five breath cycles, as in level 1, then switch sides.

Level 3 (Increased Load on Lumbar Spine and Rectus Abdominis, and the Obliques Are Active)

Starting position is the same as for level 1. Exhale to lift one leg into the tabletop position. Inhale while holding the position. Exhale to bring the opposite leg to the tabletop position, ensuring that the neutral position can be maintained and there is no doming of the abdomen (see photo *c*). If either happens, return to level 2 until the correct form can be achieved. Pump the arms up and down for 10 breath cycles as in level 1 and 2 (or less if unable to perform 10 cycles correctly).

Variations

1. For levels 1 and 3: To inhibit overactive hip flexors, squeeze a small ball or magic circle between the knees.
2. For level 2: To increase the challenge before moving to level 3, place a small ball under the foot of the nontabletop leg (see photo *d*).
3. For levels 2 and 3: To decrease the challenge to the core, place a large physio ball under the leg(s) for support.

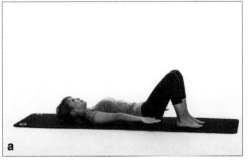

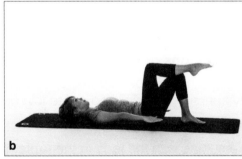

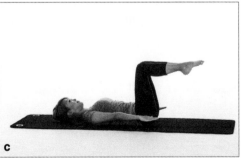

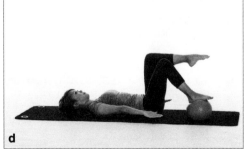

Progression

Hundred prep (p. 66) and hundred (p. 67)

Technique Tips

1. Breathe deep and long.
2. Keep the pumping motion smooth, small, and tension free. Imagine floating on a raft in a lake, tapping the surface of the water but only causing minimal ripples.
3. Avoid hyperlordosis, neck tension, bulging abdominals, and tension in the hip flexors.

HUNDRED PREP

Primary Muscles Involved

Abdominals

Objectives

Abdominal strength, trunk stabilization, and lumbo-pelvic control with an open-chain load

Indications

This exercise is a preparation for one of the classic and most well-known Pilates exercises, the hundred. It is similar to the chest lift, but with increased load on the abdominals due to the overhead position of the arms and increased challenge on the upper core due to lack of support of the neck and head.

Precautions or Contraindications

Disk pathology, osteoporosis, neck pain or pathology, acute sacroiliac joint dysfunction or pain, and acute low back pain

Instruction

Lie supine with the legs in the tabletop position and the arms overhead (see photo *a*) and then inhale to set the core. Exhale while bringing the arms down to the sides as the head, chest, and upper torso are lifted off the mat (see photo *b*). Inhale to return to the starting position.

Variations

1. To inhibit overactive hip flexors, squeeze a small ball or magic circle between the knees.
2. To remove load from the lumbar spine, place the legs over a physio ball (see photo *c*)

Progression

Hundred on the mat (p. 67), hundred on the reformer (p. 103), and hundred prep on the reformer (p. 102)

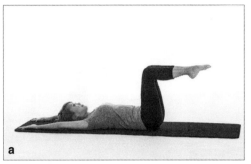
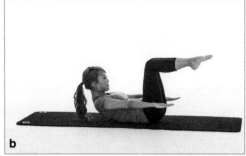
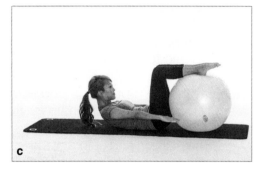

Technique Tips

1. Move the whole upper trunk and head as one unit.
2. Avoid hyperlordosis and attempt to keep the pelvis in neutral or slight posterior tilt.
3. Relax the neck and shoulders.
4. Reach toward the feet with the arms, engaging the scapular depressors.
5. The abdominals should not bulge out or dome. If it is not possible to perform the exercise without either happening, the strength and control of the core muscles is not adequate and the pre-hundred prep exercises (p. 64) should be substituted.

HUNDRED

Primary Muscles Involved

Abdominals

Objectives

Abdominal strength and lumbo-pelvic stabilization

Indications

This is a very challenging exercise that elicits isometric cocontraction of the core muscles during percussive breathing and arm movement. The long lever of the legs places a large load on the lumbar spine and hip flexors, as well as a great demand on the abdominals. The pumping motion stimulates circulation and coordination. However, besides being contraindicated for some pathologies, this exercise is too difficult and thus counterproductive for many people with lower back injuries or weakness. Therefore, I suggest starting with pre-hundred prep exercises, levels 1, 2, and 3 (p. 64), for those with lower back injuries.

Precautions or Contraindications

Disk pathology, osteoporosis, neck pain or pathology, acute sacroiliac joint dysfunction or pain, and acute low back pain

Instruction

As in hundred prep, start by lying supine with the legs in the tabletop position, arms overhead (see photo *a*). Exhale and lift the arms, head, and chest as the legs straighten and the arms are lowered to the sides of the body and parallel to the mat. Inhale to set the core and hold the position (see photo *b*). Exhale five breaths as the arms pump up and down in a small movement, then inhale for five breaths and pumps.

Note: The position and height of the legs will vary depending on hamstring flexibility and abdominal strength and control. The difficulty increases when the legs are straighter and lower.

Variations

To decrease the difficulty and strain on the lower back, the feet can be placed on the floor, in the tabletop position (as in hundred prep, photo *b*, p. 67), or supported by a physio ball (see photo *c*, hundred prep, p. 67).

Progression

Hundred on the reformer (p. 103)

Technique Tips

1. Breathe deep and long.
2. Keep the pumping motion smooth, small, and tension free. Imagine floating on a raft in a lake, tapping the surface of the water but only causing minimal ripples.
3. Avoid hyperlordosis, neck tension, bulging abdominals, and tension in the hip flexors.

MODIFIED SINGLE-LEG STRETCH (LEG SLIDES)

Primary Muscles Involved

Abdominals

Objectives

Abdominal strength and lumbo-pelvic stability

Indications

The modified single-leg stretch is a precursor to the single-leg stretch; we can start to develop abdominal strength isometrically while the legs move in a reciprocal sagittal plane leg movement, functionally similar to walking. In this version, the foot stays in contact with either the floor or a ball, decreasing load on the spine and challenge on the core. Further, the elimination of trunk flexion makes it an appropriate exercise for disk pathologies and osteoporosis. It is great for neuromuscular retraining dissociation of the legs and pelvis in a supported, stable position.

Precautions or Contraindications

Level 2 only: Acute sacroiliac joint dysfunction or pain and acute low back pain

Instruction

Lie supine with the knees bent, feet on the mat in a parallel position approximately hip-distance apart, arms straight at the sides with palms down, and pelvis in a neutral position (see photo *a*). Set the core and inhale as one foot slides out into hip and knee extension (a sock on a slick surface is helpful) (see photo *b*), then exhale to draw the leg back to the starting position. Repeat 5 to 10 times and then switch to the other leg.

Variations

To decrease the challenge, place the heel of the moving leg on a medium-size physio ball for support or decrease the range of motion to only that in which pelvic stabilization can be maintained.

Progression

Level 2: Place a small ball under one foot, and repeat the main instructions for this exercise (see photo *c*).

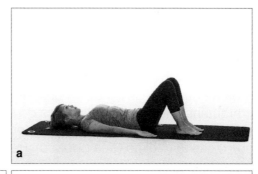

a

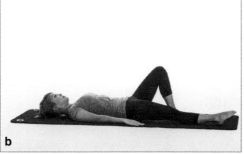

b

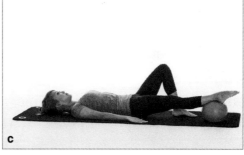

c

Technique Tips

1. Avoid an anterior tilt of the pelvis as the leg extends or a posterior tilt as the leg flexes.
2. Avoid rotation of the pelvis on the stabilizing side as the opposite leg moves in and out.
3. Imagine lengthening through the heel as the leg straightens.
4. Keep the neck and shoulders relaxed.

SINGLE-LEG STRETCH

Primary Muscles Involved

Abdominals

Objectives

Abdominal strength and lumbo-pelvic stability

Indications

This challenging exercise develops abdominal strength isometrically (trunk and pelvis are absolutely still) while the legs do the movement. Thus, lumbo-pelvic control is challenged with reciprocal open-chain sagittal plane leg movement, similar to walking. It is great for neuromuscular retraining dissociation of the legs and pelvis.

Precautions or Contraindications

Disk pathology, osteoporosis, neck pain or pathology, acute sacroiliac joint dysfunction or pain, and acute low back pain

Instruction

Lie supine with the knees bent in the tabletop position, head and chest lifted, and one hand pressing down on each knee (see photo *a*). Exhale as one leg straightens and both hands press down on the bent knee (see photo *b*). Then inhale to change legs, keeping the feet on the same horizontal plane and the legs close to midline (see photo *c*). Repeat, switching hands to the bent knee with each repetition.

Variations

To decrease the difficulty and strain on the lower back, substitute the modified single-leg stretch (leg slides) (p. 68).

Progression

Single-arm coordination on reformer (p. 106)

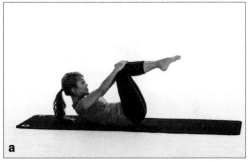

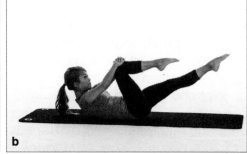

Technique Tips

1. Maintain a consistent height and a stable position of the trunk. The shoulder blades should be off the mat throughout the exercise if possible.

2. Keep the feet at the same height (approximately eye level) throughout the exercise, with the shin of the bent leg parallel to the mat.

3. Pull the bent knee in slightly closer than tabletop position, but not too close to the chest.

SHOULDER BRIDGE PREP

Primary Muscles Involved

Abdominals, back extensors, hamstrings, and gluteus maximus

Objectives

Lumbo-pelvic stabilization, hip extensor strength, development of hip dissociation, development of back extensor control, and cocontraction of core muscles

Indications

This is a great exercise for challenging lumbar stabilization as well as strengthening the glutes in a functional movement pattern. The ability to maintain height and stability of the pelvis as one leg lifts is very challenging, as well as revealing of unilateral weaknesses.

Precautions or Contraindications

Cervical disk pathology, acute back pain, and acute sacroiliac joint pathology

Instruction

Start in the up position of the pelvic curl (see pelvic curl, photo *b*, p. 57). Exhale and lift one leg up to the tabletop position, moving only at the hip joint and keeping the pelvis level (see photo *a*). Inhale and lower the leg to tap the mat (see photo *b*). Repeat 5 to 10 times with one leg and then switch sides. Complete the exercise by placing both feet on the mat and rolling down one vertebra at a time as in the pelvic curl (p. 57).

Variations

Instead of repeating the leg lift on one side for 5 to 10 repetitions, switch sides after each lift. This reciprocal movement makes the exercise more functional as well as increases the challenge to pelvic stability in the transverse plane.

Progression

1. Feet on a foam roll or ball (see photo *c*)
2. Shoulder bridge (p. 73)
3. Bottom lift on the reformer (p. 94) and variations

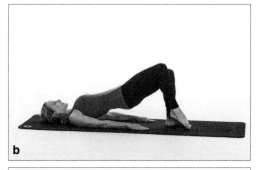

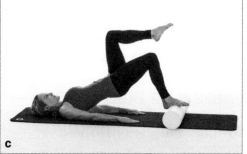

Technique Tips

1. Keep the adductors engaged to avoid splaying of the legs. A block or ball between the knees can be used if this is an issue.
2. Maintain hip extension, striving to feel a stretch in the hip flexor of the supporting leg.
3. Maintain 90 degrees of knee flexion in the moving leg.
4. The pelvis should remain stable and level, with minimal weight shift as the leg lifts.
5. Visualize a straight line of energy that runs from the shoulders, through the hips, to the knees.

SHOULDER BRIDGE

Primary Muscles Involved

Abdominals, back extensors, hamstrings, and gluteus maximus

Objectives

Lumbo-pelvic stabilization, hip extensor strength, development of hip dissociation, development of back extensor control, cocontraction of core muscles, and increased hamstring flexibility

Indications

The indications are the same as for shoulder bridge prep (p. 71), but this exercise is even more challenging. Rather than the leg lifting in a controlled manner with a bent knee, this is a dynamic swinging motion with increased torque due to the longer lever arm (perpendicular distance from the joint axis to the line of action) thus increasing the pelvic stabilization effort.

Precautions or Contraindications

Cervical disk pathology, acute back pain, and acute sacroiliac joint pathology

Instruction

Start in the up position of shoulder bridge prep (see photo a, page 72), then straighten the lifted leg toward the ceiling (see photo a). Exhale and lower the leg straight toward the mat with the foot plantar flexed (see photo b). Inhale and kick the leg straight back up with the foot dorsi flexed (see photo c). Repeat 5 to 10 times, then bend the knee and return to starting position. Switch legs and repeat the sequence on the other side. Complete the exercise by rolling down as in the pelvic curl.

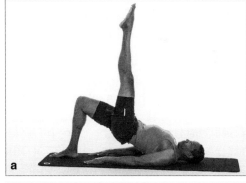

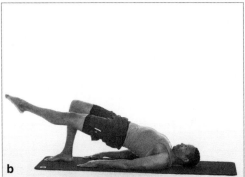

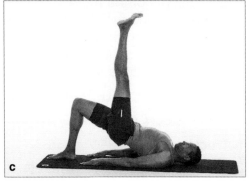

Progression

Perform the exercise with the feet on a foam roll or ball as in shoulder bridge prep.

Technique Tips

1. Maintain the pelvis in a slight posterior tilt to prevent hyperlordosis of the lumbar spine when the leg lowers.
2. Keep the adductors engaged to avoid splaying of the legs.
3. Think of the moving leg elongating on the way down, feeling a stretch across the hip flexor.
4. Actively dorsi flex the foot on the way up so that a stretch is felt on the back of the leg.
5. Keep the pelvis stable and level with minimal tipping as the leg lifts and lowers.

FRONT SUPPORT

Primary Muscles Involved

Abdominals and scapular stabilizers

Objectives

Trunk stabilization, scapular stabilization, upper body strength, and cocontraction of the abdominals and back extensors in an upper-body weight-bearing (closed-chain) position

Indications

This exercise challenges lumbo-pelvic stability in a position where the trunk is not supported; thus, skilled activation of the abdominals is needed to counteract the effect of gravity pulling the lumbar spine into extension. However, a delicate balance of the core muscles is required so that the abdominals are not overactivated, producing a posterior pelvic tilt and flexion of the spine. It is also a great way to start to build scapular stabilization strength in preparation for some of the more advanced exercises on the equipment that rely on weight-bearing function of the shoulder. It is one of my favorite exercises because although it is very challenging, the spine is not moved into contraindicated positions, so it is safe for all lumbar pathologies, assuming the patient has the required core strength to hold proper form.

Precautions or Contraindications

Shoulder, elbow, or wrist injury or severe upper body or core weakness

Instruction

From a quadruped position with the hands directly under the shoulders and fingers facing forward, establish a neutral spine and draw the shoulder blades down and back. Then inhale as one leg extends to the plank position, keeping the pelvis as still as possible (see photo *a*). Exhale and extend the other leg back into full plank position, keeping the arms and legs straight (see photo *b*). Hold this position for a few seconds while deepening the connection to the core muscles then pull the opposite knee in to touch the mat lightly. Reach that leg back to plank and slowly alternate sides.

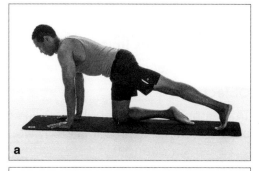

a

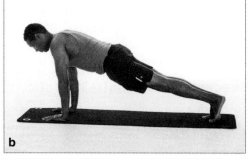

b

Variations

For those with upper extremity injuries or the inability to maintain proper form, this exercise can be modified to front support on elbows (see photo *c*). All of the same benefits are achieved, but in a more approachable position for many because it does not stress the wrists or shoulders. Electromyogram studies done by Ekstrom, Donatelli, and Carp (2007) show this exercise to be a great way to strengthen the abdominals without a lot of stress to the low back (43 percent maximum voluntary isometric contraction for rectus abdominis and 47 percent for external obliques).

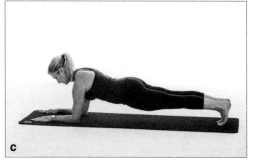

c

Progression

1. Leg pull front (p. 76)
2. Long stretch on the reformer (p. 143)

Technique Tips

1. Keep the body in a straight line from head to toe, avoiding valleys (anterior pelvic tilt or lumbar hyperlordosis) and mountains (posterior pelvic tilt or excessive lumbar flexion).
2. Maintain scapular stabilization by rooting the hands into the ground and keeping the elbows straight as the shoulder blades draw down and back (scapular adduction and depression).

LEG PULL FRONT

Primary Muscles Involved

Abdominals, scapular stabilizers, and hip extensors

Objectives

Trunk stabilization, scapular stabilization, upper body strength, cocontraction of core muscles in an upper-body weight-bearing (closed-chain) position, and hip extensor strength

Indications

The indications are the same as for front support (p. 74), with additional application for those needing to increase the strength of weak or inhibited glutes. This exercise is also helpful in teaching pelvis and hip dissociation.

Precautions or Contraindications

Shoulder, elbow, or wrist injury or severe upper body or core weakness

Instructions

Starting from the front support position, lift one leg slightly off the mat with the foot in plantar flexion. Exhale to lift the leg higher, extending at the hip without losing the neutral position of the pelvis (see photo a). Inhale to lower the leg and tap the mat (see photo b). Repeat 5 to 10 times and then switch legs.

Variations

For those with upper extremity injuries or the inability to maintain the proper form, this exercise can be modified to leg pull front on elbows (as in front support on elbows variation, photo c p. 75). All of the same benefits are achieved, but in a more approachable position for many because it does not stress the wrists or shoulders.

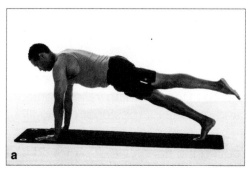 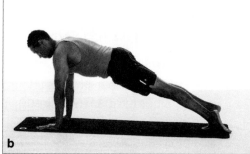

Progression

1. Shoulder push and unilateral progression (p. 146)
2. Modified balance control front (p. 147)

Technique Tips

1. Reach out through the toes of the moving leg, making the leg as straight and long as possible.
2. Keep the pelvis facing the mat and don't let the lifting leg cause the pelvis to rotate.
3. Keep the rest of the body completely still as the leg lifts, even if this means the amount of hip extension is very small. The important part of this exercise is being able to maintain the pelvic position (neutral with a bias toward a slight posterior tilt) as the leg moves up and down.
4. Press down into the mat with the hands (or elbows and forearms for leg pull front on elbows) while drawing the shoulder blades down toward the back pockets. This will ensure use of the serratus anterior and lower trapezius to keep the scapulae adducted and depressed.

SIDE BEND

Primary Muscles Involved

Oblique abdominals, quadratus lumborum, gluteus medius, and scapular stabilizers

Objectives

Abdominal oblique strength, shoulder strength, scapular stabilization, trunk stabilization, gluteus medius strength, and lateral flexion mobility

Indications

This is a great exercise for both trunk and scapular stabilization. Similar to the front support (p. 74), it can be used with all lumbar pathologies because it is performed in a neutral position. However, it is a very advanced exercise since only the feet and one arm are supporting the entire weight of the body. The scapular depressors have to work against gravity to maintain the scapula in a neutral position.

Precautions or Contraindications

Shoulder, elbow, or wrist injury; severe upper body or core weakness; and acute lumbar facet joint injury

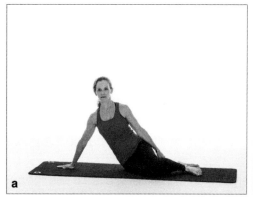

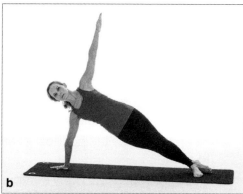

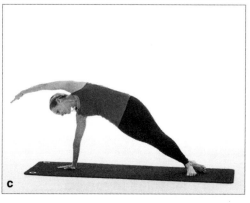

Instruction

Sit sideways on the mat with the weight on one hip. Press the palm of the supporting arm into the mat with the fingers pointing away from the body. Bend the legs and place the top foot in front of the bottom foot. Rest the top arm along the side of the body (see photo *a*). Inhale as the pelvis lifts away from the mat, straightening both legs and raising the top arm to 90 degrees of shoulder abduction (see photo *b*). Exhale as the pelvis lifts higher into a laterally flexed position and the top arm reaches overhead (see photo *c*). Inhale to return to the previous position, then exhale to lower down to the starting position. Repeat 5 to 10 times, then switch to the other side.

Variations

1. For those with upper extremity injuries or the inability to maintain the proper form, this exercise can be modified to side bend on elbow (see photo *d*). All of the same benefits are achieved, but in a more approachable position for many because it does not stress the wrists or shoulders. The side bend on elbow variation (commonly referred to as side bridge by physical therapists) has been called an optimal exercise for trunk stability because high electromyogram activity is seen in the gluteus medius (74 percent maximum voluntary isometric contraction), external obliques (69 percent), lumbar multifidi (44 percent), longissimus (40 percent), and rectus abdominis (34 percent) (Ekstrom, Donatelli, and Carp 2007).

2. For both side bend and side bend on elbow, to make the exercise easier, either keep both knees bent and in contact with (or supported by) the ground (see photo *e*), or bend the top knee and place the foot flat on the mat in front of the body (see photo *f*).

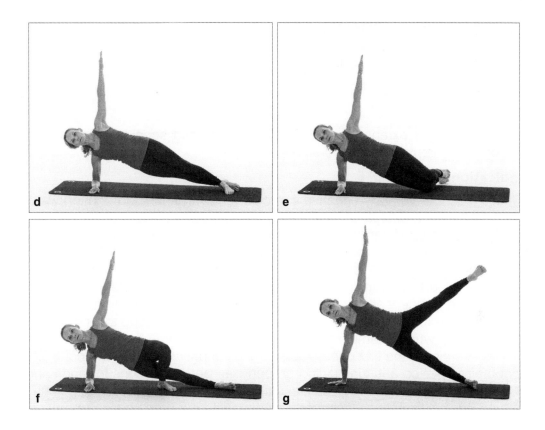

Progression

For both side bend and side bend on elbow, increase the challenge by stacking the top foot on top of the bottom foot or lift the top leg toward the ceiling so that the body is in a star position (see photo *g*).

Technique Tips

1. Initiate the movement from the oblique abdominal muscles by imagining pulling the body up with the side body rather than pushing up with the legs.
2. Maintain abdominal engagement and core connection throughout the exercise.
3. Keep the legs squeezing together.
4. Use the gluteus medius to lift the lower side of the pelvis up.
5. The body should be in one line from head to toes, as if squeezed in between two panes of glass.
6. Keep the scapular stabilizers engaged by drawing the shoulder blades down and back throughout the exercise.

BASIC BACK EXTENSION

Primary Muscles Involved

Back extensors and abdominals

Objectives

Strengthen back extensors, develop abdominal and scapular control, and cocontract core muscles

Indications

This is a simple yet very effective exercise for strengthening the often weak back extensor muscles as well as further developing control of the core muscles (both upper and lower). In prone, our back is not supported by the ground as it is in supine, and we have to counteract gravity to lift. Thus, skilled activation and coordination of the upper and lower core muscles, as well as the more superficial trunk muscles, is required. Each intervertebral segment is activated sequentially from top to bottom, thereby preventing the shear forces often experienced in the low back as most people tend to hinge at the lumbar spine when attempting back extension.

This exercise is the first one I teach to cervical patients once I am confident that their upper core is functioning properly, as per instructions for engaging the upper core in chapter 4 (p. 42), and that their muscles are ready to be challenged against gravity. I recommend starting with the prep version (p. 80)—a variation of this exercise.

Precautions or Contraindications

Spondylolisthesis, stenosis (if painful), and acute neck pain

Instruction

Lie prone with the forehead resting on a small (1 inch; 2.54 cm) cushion or small rolled-up towel so that the cervical spine is in a neutral position. Arms are by the sides with the palms pressing in against straight legs and drawing down toward plantar flexed feet (see photo *a*). Set the core muscles, both upper (chin nod) and lower (TrA or pelvic floor) as described in chapter 4. Inhale and maintain this connection as the head and upper back lift slightly off the mat, sequentially from top to bottom. Hold at the top for a couple of breath cycles (depending on ability) (see photo *b*). Exhale to lower to the starting position sequentially from bottom to top, emphasizing abdominal engagement and eccentric control of the spinal extensors. Repeat 5 to 10 times.

Variations

Prep: Use the same instructions as for the basic back extension, but do not lift the head and trunk (see photo *c*). Instead, focus on the neuromuscular

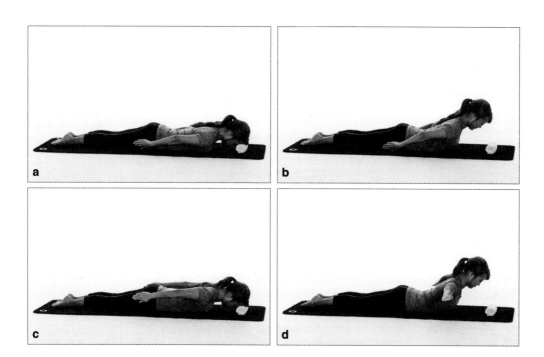

a

b

c

d

retraining of the deep neck flexors (DNF) (p. 42) and isolation of the LT muscles via reaching the arms long and lifting them slightly off the mat. This version is recommended for anyone with neck pain or cervicogenic headaches, as it begins to retrain and strengthen the cervical stabilizers without causing any of the neck tension that often results from lifting the head against gravity.

Progression

From the up position of basic back extension, reach the arms out to a *T* position while keeping the trunk lifted and stable. Hold for a couple of breath cycles, then bring the arms back to the sides and press into the thighs. Lower to the starting position and repeat 5 to 10 times (see photo *d*).

Technique Tips

1. Maintain activation of the deep neck flexors and keep the head aligned with the spine throughout the exercise.
2. Elongate the neck and imagine reaching out through the crown of the head.
3. Keep the legs together and reaching long.
4. Maintain abdominal engagement, perhaps even biasing toward a slight posterior tilt of the pelvis to protect the lower back.
5. Relax the lower body and focus on working above the waist.
6. Press the arms against the sides of the legs and reach toward the feet to ensure activation of the scapular stabilizers.

SPHINX (PREP FOR SWAN DIVE PREP)

Primary Muscles Involved

Back extensors, deep neck flexors, lower trapezius, and serratus anterior

Objectives

To retrain coactivation of the upper core (DNF, LT, and serratus anterior) and strengthen back extensors of the cervical and thoracic region

Indications

The advanced classical exercises swan dive prep and swan dive are both effective in strengthening the back extensors and maintaining a flexible spine as well as beautiful to watch when executed correctly, but they are not appropriate for most cases of spinal injury rehab; therefore, they are beyond the scope of this book. However, these versions adapted from the Australian Physiotherapy and Pilates Association (Withers and Bryant 2011) are excellent for patients with neck pain who need retraining of the upper core, as well as for clients with forward head or rounded shoulder posture. These exercises progress the retraining of the upper core described in chapter 4 (p. 42). Once the patient has learned how to stabilize the cervical region via activation of the upper core, global movements (head or arm) are integrated.

Precautions or Contraindications

Spondylolisthesis and acute neck pain

Instruction

Lie prone, propped up on forearms with elbows slightly forward of the shoulders and palms facing down. Look down at the mat so that the neck is in slight flexion (see photo *a*). Inhale and do a chin nod to activate the DNF. Exhale and spread wide across the collar bones (use the middle and lower trapezius muscles to draw the shoulders down and back by visualizing the collar bones moving apart, as opposed to rounding the upper back and shoulders forward. Inhale and lift the sternum away from the mat without moving anything else (protraction) to activate the serratus anterior. While maintaining this position and the engagement of the DNF, LT, and serratus anterior, inhale while slowly articulating one vertebra at a time, lengthening through the top of the head until looking forward (the lower cervical spine is now in slight extension) (see photo *b*). Exhale as this articulation is reversed to the starting position. Release everything and repeat the sequence three to five times.

Variations

Perform the exercise positioned in quadruped over a physio ball. The hands and knees must have firm contact with the mat (see photo *c*). This version is great for patients with lumbar spondylolisthesis, hyperlordosis, or pain when in a prone position. The cue to activate the serratus anterior in this position is to simply, "float the sternum up away from the ball."

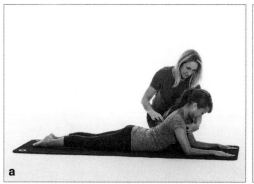

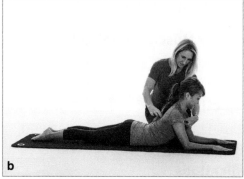

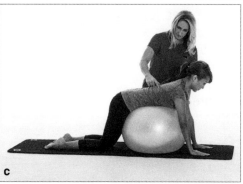

Technique Tips

1. Tactile cueing to activate the lower trapezius (the thumb and first finger of one hand at inferior angles of the scapulae) and serratus anterior (the thumb and first finger of the other hand on the patient's sternum) is very helpful for this exercise. Refer to the instructions in chapter 4 (p. 42) for setting the upper core (DNF, LT, and serratus anterior).

2. Avoid jutting the chin forward by maintaining the chin nod throughout the exercise.

3. Elongate through the neck by reaching the crown of the head away from the tailbone, rather than thinking of simply lifting the head.

4. Keep the lower core engaged throughout the exercise.

5. Keep the superficial neck muscles (sternocleidomastoid, scalenes, and upper trapezius) relaxed.

GOALPOST (PREP FOR SWAN DIVE PREP)

Primary Muscles Involved

Back extensors, deep neck flexors, and lower trapezius

Objectives

Retrain the upper core muscles and strengthen the back extensors

Indications

The indications are the same as for the sphinx (p. 82). This exercise is a modification of the classic swan dive prep exercise for patients with cervical pathologies who need retraining of the upper core. It is a great exercise for improving posture.

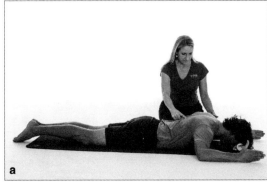

Precautions or Contraindications

Spondylolisthesis or acute neck pain

Instruction

Lie prone with the forehead resting on a small cushion or rolled-up towel

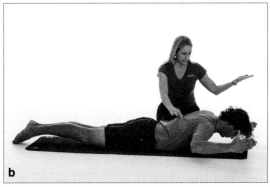

so that the cervical spine is in the neutral position. Arms should be in a goalpost position (90 degrees shoulder abduction and 90 degrees elbow flexion) with the thumbs facing the ceiling, legs together and straight with plantar flexed feet (see photo a). Inhale and do a chin nod. Then exhale and spread wide across the collar bones, drawing the shoulder blades down and back. Inhale and lift the entire upper quarter to hover off the floor, maintaining DNF and LT engagement (see photo b). Hold for a couple of breath cycles, then lower to the starting position.

Variations

For acute neck pain or cervicogenic headaches, omit the upper torso lifting off the mat. The activation of the DNF and LT, as well as lower core connection and lifting of the arms make it a valuable retraining exercise even if the head and neck are relaxed on the mat.

Progression

1. Swimming (p. 85)
2. Modified swan on floor on wunda chair (p. 198)

Technique Tips

1. Tactile cueing is very helpful for this exercise. Follow the instructions for setting the upper core (DNF and LT) in chapter 4 (p. 42).
2. Avoid jutting the chin forward by maintaining the chin nod throughout the exercise.
3. Elongate through the neck by reaching the crown of the head away from the tailbone, rather than thinking of lifting the head.
4. Keep the lower core engaged throughout the exercise.
5. Keep the superficial neck muscles (sternocleidomastoid, scalenes, upper trapezius) relaxed.

SWIMMING

Primary Muscles Involved

Back extensors and hip extensors

Objectives

Back extensor strength, hip extensor strength, trunk stabilization, and cross-pattern coordination

Indications

This is another very effective exercise for strengthening the back extensor muscles as well as developing control of the core muscles (both upper and lower) against gravity. An added benefit here is cross-pattern coordination, making it a functional retraining exercise for activities like walking and running. As one leg and the opposite arm lift up, the trunk rotates, activating the multifidi muscles, which are so important in spinal stabilization.

Precautions or Contraindications

Spondylolisthesis, stenosis, acute neck or low back pain, or shoulder impingement syndrome

Instruction

Lie prone with the arms reaching overhead, palms down, and the legs together with feet plantar flexed. Engage the upper and lower core. Keep the head aligned with the spine while lifting the chest, arms, and legs off mat (see photo *a*). Inhale as the right arm and left leg lift, then quickly switch to lift the left arm and right leg. Continue the inhale for five changes, then do the same movement while exhaling for five changes. Continue this pattern for 10 breath cycles (see photo *b*).

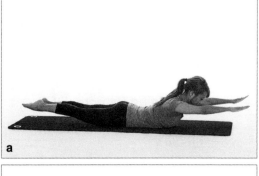

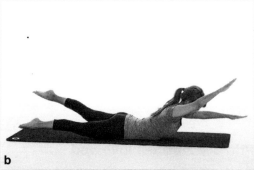

Variations

1. To make this exercise easier, allow the arm and leg that are not being lifted to remain on the mat.

2. For patients with stenosis, hyperlordosis, or pain in the prone position, place a pillow or cushion under the abdomen so that the lumbar spine is in a more neutral or even flexed position.

3. For patients with spondylolisthesis perform the exercise in quadruped position, using the abdominals to keep the pelvis in a slight posterior tilt. The leg should not lift any higher than trunk level, avoiding lumbar extension (see photo c).

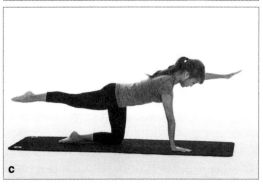

Technique Tips

1. Avoid shoulder elevation by drawing the shoulder blades down toward the back pockets.

2. Maintain trunk and pelvic stability throughout the exercise.

3. Instead of big movements, think about reaching the limbs long and straight. Keep the range of motion of the arms and legs small, like a flutter kick when swimming.

4. Avoid the chin thrusting forward and the pelvis anteriorly tilting by keeping both the upper and lower core engaged throughout.

6

Reformer Exercises

Of all the Pilates equipment, the reformer offers the most variety of movements, and it accommodates movement throughout the full range of motion (ROM) as adjustments can be made according to patient size or limitations. Exercises done on the reformer range from fundamental to extremely advanced and include all positions: supine, prone, sitting, kneeling, and standing. We can even get cardiovascular exercise and plyometrics with use of the jump board attachment. From a rehab standpoint, I prefer working on the reformer, especially in the initial stages of rehab or prehab, because it provides a wonderful viewpoint for both the client and the instructor from which to observe alignment and muscular patterning. It also allows a patient to be positioned in such a way as to help remove gravity from the equation, allowing for earlier progressive load bearing.

Similar to the mat exercises in the previous chapter, each reformer exercise is described with detailed instruction, primary muscles involved, objectives, indications, and precautions or contraindications, variations and progressions as appropriate, and technique tips for correct execution. In addition, suggested spring resistance is given. As introduced in chapter 4, the spring tension on the reformer is as follows:

Extra light= half spring (25 to 50 percent)

Light = one to one and a half springs

Medium = two to three springs

Heavy = three and a half to four springs

Extra heavy = four and a half to five springs

Some manufacturers color code individual springs to designate the resistance:

Yellow = quarter or extra light

Blue = half or light

Red = one or medium

Green = one and a half or heavy

The exercise instructions are written in a voice such that a professional can instruct his or her patient or client, and such that the directions can be followed by the practitioner him or herself. I recommend that anyone who does not have experience with Pilates works with a certified instructor to practice the exercises, both in the role of the client and of the teacher, before applying them in a rehabilitation practice. This is essential in being able to provide a safe and effective exercise program.

FOOTWORK

Primary Muscles Involved

Hamstrings, quadriceps, and gastrocnemius (calf raise and prances positions)

Objectives

Hip extensor strength, knee extensor strength, warm-up, cocontraction of core muscles in a lower body weight-bearing (closed-chain) position, and lumbo-pelvic stability, as well as hip adductor strength and control and increased ROM of the hip joints (open *V* positions), foot and ankle strength and control (parallel toes, *V*-position toes, open *V* toes, calf raises, and prances), stretch of the plantar flexors (prances and prehensile), and stretch of the foot intrinsics (prehensile)

Indications

Footwork is great as a warm-up as it uses the larger muscle groups, is attainable for almost everyone, and provides a great way to get accustomed to the equipment. It is also a great place to teach patients to focus on both the concentric and eccentric contraction as the legs straighten and bend. With proper cueing, we can emphasize the eccentric phase, so important in functional activities but so often overlooked during strengthening exercises. This exercise reinforces natural upright alignment of the body, but in a zero-gravity position, making it very valuable for patients who have difficulty standing or bearing weight due to an injury or balance issue. We can still work on upright posture and alignment without stressing the joints or worrying about balance. In addition, the footwork offers the teacher and student a great deal of information regarding strength, flexibility, stabilization, alignment, and movement patterning. The core remains constant while the musculature of the lower body is challenged in subtly different ways by simply changing the position of the feet.

Precautions or Contraindications

1. For lower extremity post-op conditions in which knee or hip flexion must be limited, foot bar or stopper adjustments can be made.
2. Certain neurological conditions or acute foot or ankle injuries may need to use the jump board attachment rather than the foot bar to provide more stability.
3. For patients who are sensitive to neck or shoulder compression (shoulder impingement syndrome, thoracic outlet syndrome, or acute neck pain), the pressure of the shoulder rests may increase tension in the neck and shoulders. Padding can be used or the spring tension reduced.

Resistance

Medium to heavy to extra heavy (depending on the objective). To emphasize core stabilization use a lighter spring setting. For increasing strength of the leg muscles or when the objective is increased load, use a heavier resistance.

Instruction

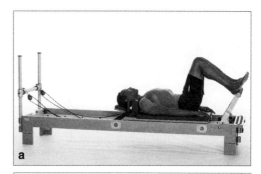

a

Lie supine in a neutral pelvis position on the reformer with the head comfortably on the headrest, feet on the foot bar (in various positions, described in the following subsections). The arms should be relaxed by the sides with the palms facing down and the shoulders lightly touching the shoulder rests. Set the core (see photo a). Exhale as the legs press out to full extension while maintaining stability in the rest of the body (see photo b). Inhale to return the carriage to the stopper, flexing the knees and hips.

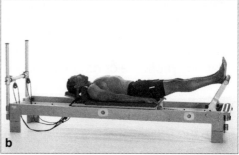

b

In BASI Pilates, the footwork is done in a particular sequence on each piece of equipment. The entire sequence is listed in order in the following subsections. Though each foot position is valuable, in the interest of time I often do only the positions I feel are most beneficial for the specific needs of the patient.

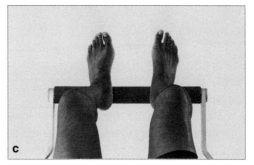

c

Parallel Heels

Place the heels approximately hip-width apart on the foot bar, with the legs parallel (as shown in photo c). This position allows us to focus on alignment and use of the legs while initially taking out the complex alignment of the foot, thus allowing the movement to occur primarily in the ankle, knee, and hip. Also, weight bearing on the heel makes it easier to connect with the hamstrings when extending the hip.

Technique tip for this position: Keep the feet partially dorsi flexed and still, as if standing on the floor.

Parallel Toes

Place the toes approximately hip width apart on the foot bar, legs parallel (see photos d and e). The toe position is more challenging than the heel position because more joints are involved, and the amount of resistance increases due to the added height of the foot.

Technique tips for this position: There is a tendency to maximally plantar flex, which results in a rocking back and forth on the ball of the foot, eliminating the ankle as the pivot point. The foot should remain active, pivoting at the ankle joint and maintaining a constant degree of plantar flexion throughout the movement (the maximum amount possible when the knees are fully extended). To cue this, place your hands on the plantar surface of the client's heels with the verbal cue to keep the pressure constant throughout the movement.

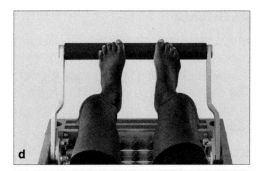

V-Position Toes

From the parallel toes position, simply bring the heels together without adjusting the width between the feet (see photo *e*). The degree of hip external rotation should not be more than 30 degrees, forming a small *V* with the feet. This is a classic Pilates position similar to a military stance.

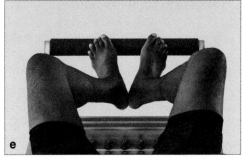

Technique tips for this position: Imagine straightening the legs and squeezing them together at the same time, as if holding a big ball between the legs. Keep the heels still while squeezing them together.

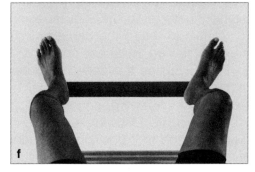

Open V Heels

Place the heels at the outside of the foot bar to form a wide *V* position with the hips externally rotated and the knees aligned over the second and third toes (see photo *f*). The wide positions are not from the classic Pilates repertoire but offer valuable benefits because the hip joint is challenged in a position of hip abduction and external rotation that is out of many people's comfort zone. To maintain optimal function of the hip joint, it is imperative to keep this ROM. These wide positions are particularly good for dancers and other athletes in developing functional strength needed.

Technique tips for this position: Imagine straightening the legs and simultaneously squeezing them together and focus on engaging the hip adductors. When the knees bend, visualize them reaching out to the sides of the body along a constant diagonal energy line. Keep the feet partially dorsi flexed and still, as if standing on the floor.

Open *V* Toes

Place the toes at the outside of the foot bar to form a wide *V* position, hips externally rotated with the knees aligned over the second and third toes (see photo *g*). This is the most complex position in the footwork because it requires a lot of control of the hip, knee, ankle, and foot. It offers the most stretch in the hip joint and a unique angle of pull for the hamstrings and quads.

Technique tips for this position: As in parallel toes, there is a tendency to maximally plantar flex. The foot should remain active, pivoting at the ankle joint and maintaining a constant degree of plantar flexion throughout the movement (the maximum amount possible when the knees are fully extended). Tactilely cue for this as in parallel toes.

Calf Raises

Start with the toes on the foot bar approximately hip-width apart, legs parallel and straight. The foot should be aligned in the subtalar neutral posi-

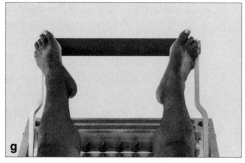

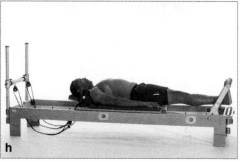

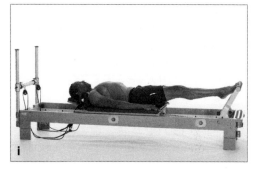

tion, avoiding excessive supination or pronation. Inhale to lower the heel slowly under the foot bar, and actively dorsi flex at the bottom (see photo *h*). Exhale to push the foot bar away from the body as the feet rise up into maximum plantar flexion (see photo *i*). This is an exceptional exercise for increasing function, ROM, and strength of the foot, and it allows focus on awareness and correction of foot alignment.

Technique tips for this position: Use full ROM of the ankle. Focus on getting as tall as possible on the up phase, and then lower the heels slowly rather than letting them drop (to maximize eccentric contraction).

Prances

Start in the same position as for calf raises (see photo *i*). Dorsi flex one foot and plantar flex the other simultaneously, alternating side to side. In addition to the benefits listed in calf raises, there is potential for a great calf stretch, which can be enhanced by the manual assist of pulling on the patient's heel (see photo *j*).

Technique tips for this position: Be sure to hit the position of maximal plantar flexion in between side switches to achieve a sense of height and elongation. Maintain a stable pelvis throughout the movement.

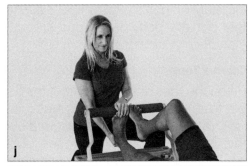

Single-Leg Heel

Start as in parallel heels (see photo *c*, page 89), but bring one leg to the tabletop position (see photo *k*). This allows each leg to work independently without relying on the other. Alignment issues and weaknesses can be easily detected. The single-leg versions are extremely valuable for injuries and post-op conditions as the stronger leg tends to dominate in the bilateral positions. In general, exercising one leg at a time increases the challenge for the core muscles to effectively keep the pelvis stable.

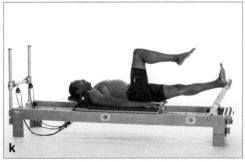

Technique tips for this position: Keep both the tabletop leg and the heel of the dorsi flexed working foot absolutely still. To help stay stable and balanced, imagine that both feet are on the bar

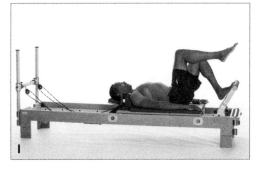

and pushing evenly through both feet, just as in the bilateral version.

Single-Leg Toe

Start as in parallel toes (see photo *d*, p. 90), but bring one leg to the tabletop position (see photo *l*). This is the most challenging position of the footwork exercises in terms of load.

Technique tips for this position: Keep both the tabletop leg and the heel of the working foot absolutely still. The tactile cue of placing one hand on the client's heel with the instruction to maintain constant pressure (as in parallel toes) is very effective. To help stay stable and balanced, the client should imagine that both feet are on the bar and pushing evenly through both feet, just as in the bilateral version.

Prehensile

Place the balls of the feet on the bar approximately hip-width apart with the legs parallel. Wrap the front part of the foot and toes around the bar and press the heels down. Exhale to straighten the legs while pushing the heels farther under the bar (see photo m). Inhale and continue pushing the heels under the bar as the knees bend and the carriage is returned to the stopper. This is a great exercise for stretching the intrinsic muscles of the foot, as well as recruiting the arch-supporting muscles for clients who overpronate.

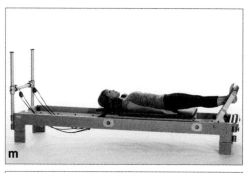

Technique tips for this position: Keep the toes spread out instead of clenched together. Imagine a bird wrapping its feet around a branch. Reach the heels under the foot bar throughout the movement to maximize the calf stretch.

Variations

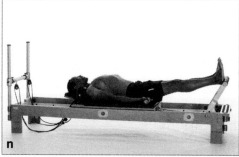

Patients with rounded shoulders or neck tension can hold a dowel under the hips with the palms facing up. This encourages external rotation of the shoulders, as well as engagement of the lower trapezius (LT) and latissimus dorsi (see photo n).

Progression

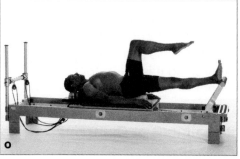

1. To increase core stability challenge, the series can be performed on a half foam roll (see photo o) or even a full foam roll.
2. To emphasize quadriceps strengthening, add a pumping series with any of these positions: parallel heels, parallel toes, V-position toes, open V heels, open V toes, single-leg heel, single leg toe. After completion of 10 repetitions, hold a mid-range position and do small, quick pumps for about 10 repetitions. After the last pump, press all the way to full extension and then return the carriage to the stopper.

Technique Tips

1. Initiate the movement from the sit bones. This elicits an emphasis on the hamstrings to counteract the overpowering quality of the quads.
2. Visualize a rubber band connecting the heels to the sit bones. As the leg straightens, the band stretches, creating a strong pull between the heels and sit bones. As the leg bends, resist the movement as if trying to keep the leg straight. This internal resistance increases the work in the muscles, maximizing the eccentric contraction.

3. Straighten the legs completely, focusing on the cocontraction of the quadriceps and the hamstrings.

4. Maintain a neutral pelvis position (or appropriate pelvic position for a specific condition) throughout the series.

5. Use the ankle as the pivot point of the movement.

BOTTOM LIFT

Primary Muscles Involved

Abdominals, hamstrings, gluteus maximus, and back extensors

Objectives

Mobilization of the spine and pelvic region, spinal articulation, hamstring control, hip extensor strength, pelvic and lumbar stabilization, and recruitment and cocontraction of the core muscles

Indications

This is basically the same exercise as the pelvic curl (p. 57), but it is much more challenging on the reformer because the movement of the carriage adds the element of instability. It takes a great deal of lumbo-pelvic stability and hip extensor control to be able to lift the hips up without moving the carriage. With the balls of the feet placed on the bar, it also takes a lot of foot and ankle control, so it is great for developing ankle stability after an ankle sprain. The height of the bar makes the available hip extension ROM greater than it is for the pelvic curl.

Precautions or Contraindications

Contraindications include acute lumbar disk pathology or osteoporosis (due to the deep lumbar flexion), cervical disk pathologies, cervicogenic headaches, or acute neck pain (due to the amount of cervical flexion and compression in this exercise). Use caution and perhaps extra padding on the shoulder rests with shoulder impingement syndrome and thoracic outlet syndrome.

Resistance

Medium

Instruction

Lie supine on the carriage with the headrest down, knees bent, the balls of the feet placed on the foot bar, and legs parallel approximately hip-width apart (see photo *a*). Exhale to draw the abdominals in and articulate the spine up, one vertebra at a time (see photo *b*). Inhale and pause at the top, then exhale to articulate the spine back down to the carriage. The movement of the carriage should be minimal.

Variations

1. For lumbar disk pathologies and osteoporosis, omit the deep lumbar flexion and maintain the spine and pelvis in a neutral position as they are lifted.
2. To make it easier, place the heels on the foot bar or use heavier resistance (more resistance provides more support, less instability).
3. Place a ball or block between the knees to promote more adductor engagement.

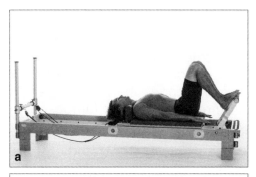
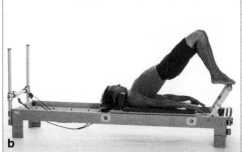

Progression

1. Bottom lift with extension (p. 95)
2. Perform the exercise unilaterally with one foot on the bar and the other leg in the tabletop position (as in photo *c*, p. 96).

Technique Tips

1. Align the feet, keeping the heels still throughout the exercise.
2. Keep the legs parallel and adductors engaged; using a ball between the knees helps.
3. To minimize the movement of the carriage and keep it as close to the stopper as possible; think of lifting up instead of pressing out.
4. Maximize lumbar flexion as the spine lifts off the mat by pulling the pubic bone towards the head (posteriorly tilting the pelvis). Once the tailbone lifts, continue peeling one vertebra at a time off the carriage as if peeling a banana.
5. Visualize the lowering of the spine like a Slinky spring toy going down steps, deliberately placing one vertebra at a time. This will help to achieve maximum articulation and spinal mobility.

BOTTOM LIFT WITH EXTENSION

Primary Muscles Involved

Abdominals, hamstrings, gluteus maximus, and back extensors

Objectives

Mobilization of the spine and pelvic region, spinal articulation, hamstring strength and control, hip extensor strength, pelvic and lumbar stabilization, and recruitment and cocontraction of the core muscles

Indications

The indications for this exercise are the same as for bottom lift, but the addition of extending the legs further challenges the hamstrings and requires even more lumbo-pelvic stabilization.

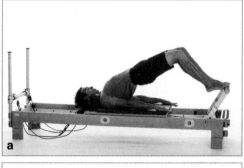

Precautions or Contraindications

Same as for bottom lift (p. 94)

Resistance

Medium

Instruction

Set up and articulate the spine up as in bottom lift (see photo b, p. 95). After the pause at the top, exhale as the legs press into extension (see photo a), then inhale to bend the knees and bring the carriage back to the stopper, keeping the hips lifted and even (see photo b). Repeat 5 to 10 times, then articulate the spine down to the starting position on an exhale.

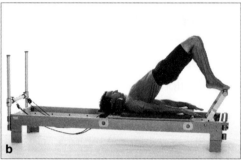

Variations

1. For clients with lumbar disk pathologies and osteoporosis, omit the deep lumbar flexion and maintain the spine and pelvis in a neutral position as they are lifted.

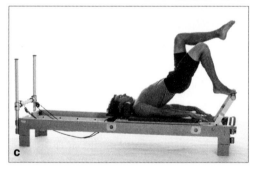

2. To make it easier, place the heels on the foot bar or use heavier resistance to increase stability.
3. Place a ball or block between the client's knees to promote more adductor engagement.

Progression

Perform the exercise with one leg in the tabletop position (see photo c).

Technique Tips

1. Keep the knees unlocked. Do not fully extend the legs, as this can strain the lower back.
2. When returning the carriage to the stopper, maintain a strong diagonal line of energy from the shoulders, through the hips, to the knees.

3. The pelvis tends to drop as the carriage comes in, so focus on keeping the hips extended and the pelvis lifted to the same height throughout the exercise.
4. Keep the heels still, legs parallel, and adductors engaged.

ARMS SUPINE SERIES

SUPINE ARM EXTENSION

Primary Muscles Involved

Latissimus dorsi

Objectives

This exercise is done to strengthen the shoulder extensors and develop trunk and scapular stabilization and scapulohumeral rhythm. The simple act of holding the legs in the tabletop position strengthens and increases the endurance of the abdominals and hip flexors.

Indications

Besides strengthening and toning the arms, the arms supine series challenges the core stabilizers and emphasizes development of a rhythmic coordination of the shoulder stabilizers (specifically the LT and serratus anterior) with the muscles that move the shoulder. This series is particularly valuable for patients because it places the body in a safe, comfortable, non–weight-bearing position in which arm and shoulder strength can be developed while maintaining trunk stabilization. Further, the entire series is done below 90 degrees of shoulder flexion, which is good for patients with painful conditions such as impingement syndrome, in which lifting the arm higher than shoulder height is often contraindicated. It is also effective in increasing the active ROM of the glenohumeral joint.

Precautions or Contraindications

None

Resistance

Light to medium

Instruction

Lie supine in a neutral pelvis position, with legs in the tabletop position, arms perpendicular to the carriage, shoulders stable with hands holding the straps or the handles and palms facing the carriage (see photo *a*). Exhale and initiate the movement from the core as the arms float straight down to the sides of the body (see photo *b*). Inhale and return to the starting position.

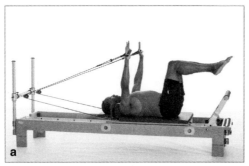 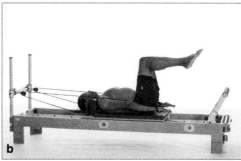

Variations

1. For patients who do not have the strength or endurance to tolerate or maintain the tabletop position, modify in one or more of the following ways:

   a. Pull the knees into the chest.

   b. Cross one ankle over the other, supporting the symptomatic leg with the opposite leg.

   c. Place a ball between the knees to increase activation of the adductors and pelvic floor muscles, thereby inhibiting overactivity of the hip flexors and decreasing strain on the lower back.

2. Patients with limited shoulder ROM as in adhesive capsulitis should work in the available pain-free range only.

3. If the goal is to increase shoulder active ROM (for example, a post-op rotator cuff surgery patient), move the body toward the foot bar so that there is space between the shoulders and shoulder rests (or remove the shoulder rests if possible on your reformer) so that they do not impede shoulder joint mobility.

Technique Tips

1. Maintain the core connection and scapular stabilization by engaging the abdominal muscles and pulling the shoulder blades into the back pockets.

2. Maintain consistent tension in the straps throughout the movement.

3. Use a smooth and even movement during both concentric and eccentric phases.

4. Keep the arms straight without placing excessive force on the elbow (don't lock out).

5. Use the arms as if they were large fins, pushing against water and propelling the body through it.

6. Keep the arms at shoulder height and below (unless the objective is to increase ROM).

SUPINE ARM ADDUCTION

Primary Muscles Involved

Latissimus dorsi

Objectives

Same as for supine arm extension (p. 97)

Indications

The indications for this exercise are the same as for supine arm extension.

Precautions or Contraindications

None

Resistance

Light to medium

Instruction

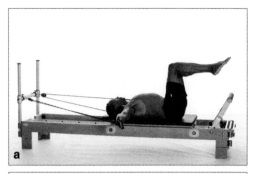

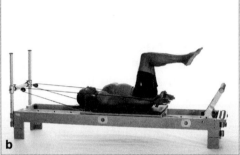

Lie supine in a neutral pelvis position with legs in the tabletop position, arms out to side in a *T* position (90 degrees shoulder abduction), shoulders stable with the hands holding the straps or the handles and palms facing the body (see photo *a*). Exhale to adduct the arms to the sides of the body (see photo *b*). Inhale to return to the starting position.

Variations

The variations for this exercise are the same as for supine arm extension (p. 97).

Technique Tips

The tips for this exercise are the same as for supine arm extension (p. 97).

SUPINE ARM CIRCLES

Primary Muscles Involved

Latissimus dorsi

Objectives

Same as for supine arm extension (p. 97), as well as to improve shoulder joint mobility

Indications

The indications for this exercise are the same as for supine arm extension. This exercise is great for patients with restricted shoulder ROM (arthritis, adhesive capsulitis, post-op rotator cuff repair).

Precautions or Contraindications

None

Resistance

Light to medium

Instruction

This exercise is simply a combination of arm extension and arm adduction. Lie supine in a neutral pelvis position, legs in the tabletop position, arms straight by sides, shoulders stable with hands holding the straps or the handles and palms facing the carriage (see photo *a*). Inhale to lift the arms to shoulder height (see photo *b*) then open out to a *T* position (see photo *c*). Exhale to adduct the arms to the sides of the body, rotating the palms to face the carriage and return to the starting position (this is referred to as up circles). Repeat the movement 5 to 10 times and then reverse direction for down circles.

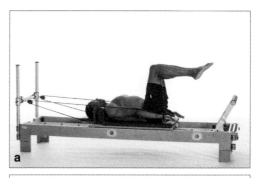

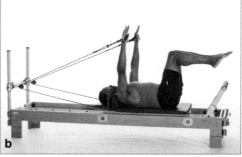

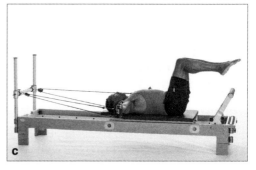

Variations

The variations for this exercise are the same as for supine arm extension (p. 97).

Technique Tips

1. The technique tips for supine arm extension (p. 97) can all be applied in this exercise.
2. Strive to keep the movement fluid, yet define exact points at the end range, as if drawing a continuous elliptical shape on the ceiling.
3. As long as there are no ROM restrictions, draw the pattern as large as possible to achieve maximum ROM of the glenohumeral joint.

TRICEPS

Primary Muscles Involved

Triceps

Objectives

Elbow extensor strength, trunk development, and scapular stabilization

Indications

The indications for this exercise are the same as for supine arm extension (p. 97).

Precautions or Contraindications

None

Resistance

Light to medium

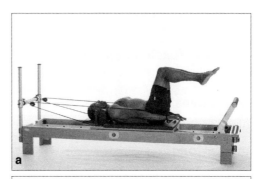

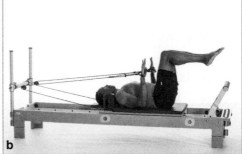

Instruction

Lie supine in a neutral pelvis position, legs in the tabletop position, arms straight by the sides, and shoulders stable with hands holding the straps or the handles and palms facing the carriage (see photo *a*). Inhale to bend the elbows (see photo *b*) and exhale to straighten the elbows.

Variations

The variations for this exercise are the same as for supine arm extension (p. 97).

Technique Tips

1. Press the arms into the sides of the body throughout the movement to assist in keeping the shoulders stable and maintaining good alignment.
2. Keep the upper arms still.
3. Keep the wrists in a neutral position.
4. Keep the arms parallel to the floor and in line with the shoulders as opposed to pushing down into the carriage with the elbows.
5. Imagine propelling oneself through water with only the forearms.
6. Keep the trunk and legs stable.

HUNDRED PREP

Primary Muscles Involved

Abdominals

Objectives

Abdominal strength, shoulder extensor strength, and lumbo-pelvic stabilization

Indications

This exercise is a preparation for one of the classic and most well-known Pilates exercises, the hundred. In essence, it is a chest lift with resistance.

Precautions or Contraindications

Disk pathology, osteoporosis, neck pain or pathology, acute sacroiliac joint dysfunction or pain, or acute low back pain

Resistance

Light to medium

Instruction

Lie supine on the reformer with legs in the tabletop position, arms perpendicular to the carriage, and hands in the straps or handles while maintaining slight tension. Ideally, the spine should be in the neutral position, but if appropriate, allow for a slight posterior tilt of the pelvis (see photo *a*). Inhale to set the core and then exhale, bringing the arms down to the sides as the head, chest, and upper torso lift up (see photo *b*). Inhale to return to the starting position.

Variations

To inhibit overactive hip flexors, squeeze a small ball or magic circle between the knees.

Progression

1. Hundred prep with extension: as the head, chest, and torso lift up, add extension of the legs. As the body lowers, the legs return to the tabletop

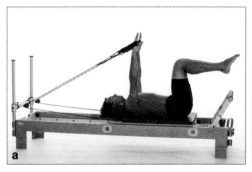 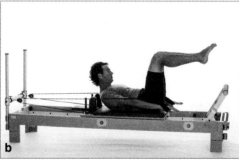

position. This increases the load on the trunk, thereby making it more challenging to maintain pelvic-lumbar stability.

2. Hundred (p. 103).

Technique Tips

1. Move the whole upper trunk and head as one unit, keeping the head aligned with the spine.
2. Avoid hyperlordosis and attempt to keep the pelvis in a neutral position or slight posterior tilt.
3. Relax the neck and shoulders.
4. Reach toward the feet with the arms, engaging the scapular depressors.
5. Do not allow the abdominals to bulge out or dome.
6. For the hundred prep with extension progression, extend the legs long, reaching out through pointed toes. The level of difficulty can be controlled by the height of the extended legs (higher is easier).

HUNDRED

Primary Muscles Involved

Abdominals

Objectives

Abdominal strength, integration of abdominals and shoulder extensors, lumbo-pelvic stabilization, stimulation of circulation and deep breathing

Indications

This is a very challenging exercise that elicits isometric cocontraction of the core muscles during percussive breathing and isotonic arm work. The long lever of the legs places a large load on the lumbar spine and hip flexors, as well as a great demand on the abdominals. The pumping motion stimulates circulation and coordination. However, besides being contraindicated for some pathologies, this exercise is too difficult and thus counterproductive for many people with lower back injuries or weakness.

Precautions or Contraindications

Disk pathology, osteoporosis, neck pain or pathology, acute sacroiliac joint dysfunction or pain, or acute low back pain

Instruction

Lie supine on the reformer with the legs in the tabletop position, arms perpendicular to the carriage, and the hands holding the straps or handles maintaining slight tension. Ideally the spine should be in a neutral position, but if appropriate allow for a slight posterior tilt of the pelvis (see photo a). Exhale and lift the arms, head, and chest as the legs straighten and the arms are lowered to the sides of the body, parallel to the mat (see photo b). While holding this position, exhale five times as the arms pump up and down in a small movement, then inhale during five breaths and arm pumps. Repeat this pumping and breathing sequence 10 times, then draw the legs back to the tabletop position and lower the body down to the starting position. Note that the position and height of the legs will vary depending on hamstring flexibility and abdominal strength and control, with the difficulty increasing when the legs are straighter and lower.

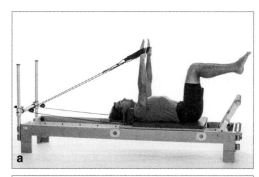

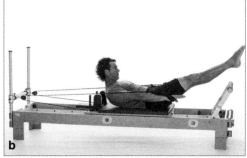

Variations

1. To decrease the difficulty and strain on the lower back, the legs can be raised toward 90 degrees of hip flexion or even placed in the tabletop position as in hundred prep (p. 102).
2. Place a ball between the knees to activate the adductors and inhibit the hip flexors.

Technique Tips

1. Breathe deep and long.
2. Keep the pumping motion smooth, small, and tension free. Imagine floating on a raft in a lake, tapping the surface of the water but causing only minimal ripples.
3. Avoid hyperlordosis, neck tension, bulging abdominals, and tension in the hip flexors.
4. Maintain consistent height throughout the exercise.
5. Keep the head aligned with the spine and the eyes looking forward.

COORDINATION

Primary Muscles Involved

Abdominals

Objectives

Abdominal strength, lumbo-pelvic stabilization, and improved coordination of breath and movement

Indications

This exercise presents both an isometric and an isotonic challenge to the abdominals, as well as a huge challenge of coordination. It is another great exercise for neuromuscular retraining of the dissociation of the legs while the core remains engaged and the pelvis remains still.

Precautions or Contraindications

Disk pathology, osteoporosis, neck pain or pathology, acute sacroiliac joint dysfunction or pain, or acute low back pain

Resistance

Light to medium

Instruction

Start with legs in the tabletop position and arms at 90 degrees of shoulder flexion as in hundred prep (see photo *a*, page 102). Exhale to lift the head and chest while reaching the arms down alongside the body and straightening the legs (see photo *a*). Continue exhaling as the legs open and close quickly (see photo *b*). Inhale as the legs bend to the tabletop position, then lower the trunk, head, and arms to the starting position.

Variations

For patients with disk pathology, osteoporosis, or neck pain or pathology the exercise can be performed without lifting the head and trunk.

Technique Tips

1. Draw the knees in before lowering the trunk.
2. Keep the head aligned with the spine and the eyes looking forward.
3. Do not allow the opening of the legs to be wider than the foot bar.
4. The opening and closing of the legs should be quite sharp and dynamic, but the lifting and lowering of the body should be smooth.

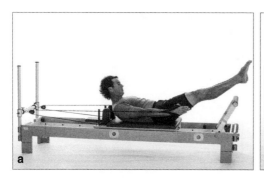 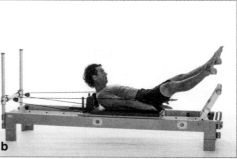

SINGLE-ARM COORDINATION

*A variation of an original exercise taught by Rael Isacowitz in the BASI Mentor Program (Isacowitz 2018).

Primary Muscles Involved

Abdominals

Objectives

Oblique abdominal strength, lumbo-pelvic stabilization primarily in the transverse plane, improved coordination, and neuromuscular training for cross-patterning

Indications

This exercise really focuses on the strength and control of the oblique abdominals. It is quite difficult in terms of coordination, as one side of the body remains still while the other moves. It is a wonderful exercise to challenge core strength and lumbo-pelvic control for patients with neck issues, disk pathology, or osteoporosis because the trunk and head remain supported in a neutral position throughout.

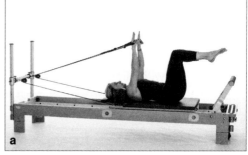

Precautions or Contraindications

Acute sacroiliac joint dysfunction or pain or acute low back pain

Resistance

Light to medium

Instruction

Lie on the carriage with the legs in the tabletop position and the arms perpendicular to the carriage (see photo a). Inhale and set the core and then exhale as the right arm reaches down alongside the body and the right leg extends straight out toward the foot bar at a 45-degree angle. The left arm and left leg should remain completely still (see photo b). Inhale to return to the starting position and repeat on the other side.

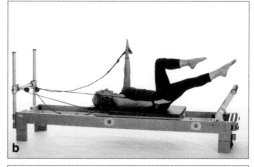

Variations

To challenge coordination and work on cross-patterning, extend the opposite arm and leg instead of the same side (see photo c). This version is easier on the obliques, but more challenging for the mind.

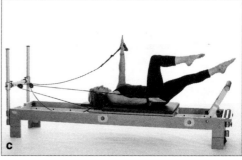

Progression

If there are no neck issues, disk pathology, or osteoporosis, the exercise can be performed with the head and chest lifted off the carriage.

Technique Tips

1. Keep the nonmoving arm very still and perpendicular to the carriage.
2. Keep the pelvis in a neutral position.
3. Be careful not to let the body shift or rotate to the side of the moving arm and leg.
4. Strive for full extension of the leg and arm with each repetition.

AB OPENINGS

*A variation of an original exercise taught by Rael Isacowitz in the BASI Mentor Program (Isacowitz 2018).

Primary Muscles Involved

Abdominals

Objectives

Abdominal strength, lumbo-pelvic stabilization, hip abduction and adduction strength and control, and improved coordination

Indications

This exercise elicits isometric cocontraction of the core muscles during lower body movement. The long lever of the legs places a large load on the lumbar spine and hip flexors, as well as a great demand on the abdominals. The opening and closing of the legs challenges coordination as well as hip strength, control, and mobility.

Precautions or Contraindications

Disk pathology, osteoporosis, neck pain or pathology, acute sacroiliac joint dysfunction or pain, or acute low back pain

Resistance

Light

Instruction

Lie supine on the carriage with the hands holding the straps or the handles, spine in a neutral position, and legs in the tabletop position (see photo a). Set the core and exhale to lift the head and torso as the legs straighten out over the foot bar along a diagonal line (approximately 60 degrees of hip flexion) and the arms reach down to the sides with the palms facing the body (see photo b). Inhale to open the legs and arms as if doing a jumping jack (see photo c) and then exhale to draw the legs and arms back in to the midline. Repeat the in-and-out movement 10 to 15 times, then return to the starting position.

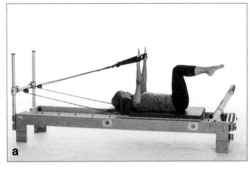

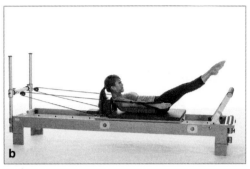

Variations

For patients who should not go into trunk flexion due to lumbar disk pathology or osteoporosis, and for those with neck pain or pathology, the exercise can be performed without lifting the head and trunk.

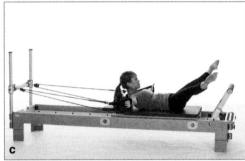

Progression

To increase the challenge on the abdominals, lower the legs to hover just above the foot bar.

Technique Tips

1. Open the legs no wider than the foot bar.
2. Relax the neck muscles.
3. Lengthen through the legs and arms.

HIP WORK SERIES (LEGS IN STRAPS)

The hip work series is a very challenging and useful series of exercises for almost anyone needing to improve pelvic stability and hip mobility. It demands more lumbo-pelvic stabilization than the footwork exercises, because the feet are in straps rather than in contact with the foot bar, making it an open-chain exercise. It is also a great way to teach the concept of hip dissociation, as smooth continuous movement of the hip joint is executed while stability of the pelvis is maintained. Imbalances in hip musculature are often the cause of lumbar, pelvic, hip, and even knee pathologies. This series addresses these imbalances; the primary muscles worked are the hip extensors, abductors, and adductors (as opposed to the often too-tight hip flexors). I have found this series to be very beneficial for patients with sacroiliac joint dysfunction.

Please note that getting into and out of this series can be dangerous. Spotting from the correct position and ensuring that the patient is in control of the straps and carriage is crucial before starting this series. I recommend standing with one leg in the well to stabilize the carriage as you assist each of the patient's

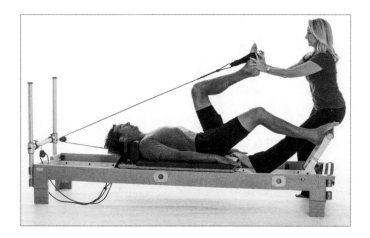

feet into the straps (see photo). Verbalize to the patient that he needs to control the movement of the carriage with the core muscles; otherwise, the carriage will come down to the stopper and the patient will go into a backwards somersault.

HIP EXTENSION

Primary Muscles Involved

Hip extensors

Objectives

Lumbo-pelvic stability, hip joint mobility, hip extensor strength, and hip dissociation

Indications

This is a great way to start the hip work series, as it reinforces pelvic stability with hip mobility (hip dissociation). It is effective in showing patients where in their range of motion they start to lose their neutral spine position and which muscles they can use to control this. The starting position elicits initiation of leg movement from the hamstrings, while at the same time giving these muscles an active stretch. It is adaptable for all, as the range can be increased or decreased according to the patient's ability or limitations.

Precautions or Contraindications

None

Resistance

Light to medium to orient the work toward stabilization. Resistance can be increased if the objective is strengthening the hip extensors.

Instruction

Lie supine in a neutral pelvis position on the carriage with the feet in the straps, arms at the sides with the palms facing down, legs straight and at a maximum of 90 degrees of hip flexion if possible (less if hamstring tightness prohibits) (see photo *a*). Exhale to lower the legs to the point where the pelvis starts to go into an anterior tilt (see photo *b*), using the deep core muscles to counteract this. Inhale to return to the starting position.

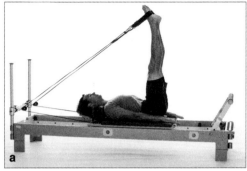

Variations

To increase the challenge and elicit adductor work, place a ball between the upper thighs or ankles.

Progression

This and the other exercises in this series can be performed lying on a half foam roll to increase the stabilization challenge.

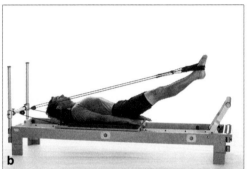

Technique Tips

1. Lengthen through the legs.
2. Keep the tailbone glued to the carriage throughout the exercise.
3. Bring the legs down toward the foot bar as far as possible without arching the back.
4. Keep the neck and shoulders relaxed.

FROG

Primary Muscles Involved

Hip adductors

Objectives

Lumbo-pelvic stabilization, hip mobility, adductor strength and control, and knee extensor control

Indications

This is a great exercise for stiff or arthritic hips and knees, sacroiliac joint pathologies, and anyone needing to develop pelvic-lumbar stabilization.

Precautions or Contraindications

Use caution with post-op total hip joint replacement patients, as the tendency is to go into >90 hip flexion when the legs pull in to the frog position.

Resistance

Light to medium for stability; heavier if the objective is adductor strength

Instruction

Lie supine on the carriage in a neutral spine position with the feet in the straps, hips flexed to 90 degrees and externally rotated, knees bent out to the sides, and heels squeezing together (see photo *a*). Exhale to straighten the legs along a diagonal line, at an approximately 45 degree angle (see photo *b*). Inhale to bend the knees and return to the starting position.

Variation

To increase the challenge, place a ball between the ankles as in hip extension, (p. 109).

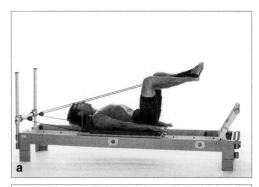

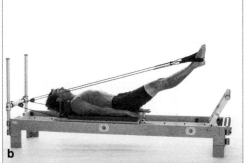

Progression

The progression for this exercise is the same as for hip extension (p. 109).

Technique Tips

1. Focus on squeezing the legs together as the knees straighten, as if holding a balloon between the legs.
2. Keep the heels glued together throughout the exercises, especially when straightening out to full knee extension.
3. Keep the pelvis stable throughout the exercise.
4. Avoid bringing the knees too close to the chest, as this can cause the tailbone to lift and it makes the exercise contraindicated for post-op total hip replacements.

DOWN CIRCLES AND UP CIRCLES

Primary Muscles Involved

Hip adductors and hip extensors

Objectives

Lumbo-pelvic stabilization; hip mobility; hip adductor, abductor, and extensor strength and control; hip dissociation; and adductor and hamstring muscle elongation

Indications

The indications for this exercise are the same as for hip extension and frog (pages 109 and 110). In addition, this is a fabulous exercise for adductor control and strength as they are forced to work isometrically, concentrically, and eccentrically. This is one of my favorite exercises for developing hip dissociation and increasing hip joint ROM.

Precautions or Contraindications

None

Resistance

Light to medium for stability, heavier if the objective is hip strength.

Instruction

Lie supine on the carriage in a neutral pelvis position with the feet in the straps, legs straight, and hips at 90 degrees of flexion (if possible without tilting the pelvis). The hips should be externally rotated and the feet should be in soft plantar flexion (see photo *a*).

Down Circles

Exhale to press the legs straight down the midline, keeping them together (see photo *b*). Inhale to open the legs and circle them around and up to the starting position (see photo *c*).

Up Circles

Start as in down circles but reverse the direction, opening the legs out before bringing them down and around, and then back up the midline to the starting position.

Progression

The progression for this exercise is the same as for hip extension (p. 109).

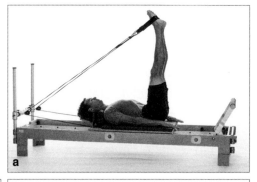

a

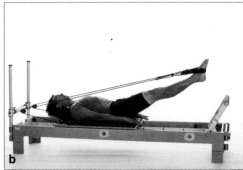

b

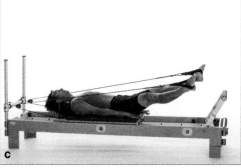

c

Technique Tips

1. Imagine drawing a circular shape on the ceiling with the feet.
2. Squeeze the legs together as they draw a line up or down the center.
3. Engage the hamstrings with the adductors as the legs are lowered down the center.
4. Maximize the contraction of the adductors when opening and closing the legs.

OPENINGS

Primary Muscles Involved

Hip adductors

Objectives

Lumbo-pelvic stabilization, hip mobility, hip adductor strength and control, hip dissociation, and adductor and hamstring muscle elongation

Indications

The indications for this exercise are the same as for frog and circles. An added benefit here is that strength and control are developed at the extremes of the hip joint's range of motion, which is very important for dancers, figure skaters, gymnasts, hockey players, and baseball catchers. This is also a wonderful exercise for those suffering from stiff hips or hip joint arthritis and for athletes who train primarily in the sagittal plane.

Precautions or Contraindications

None

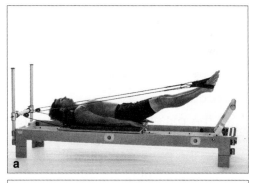

Resistance

Light to medium for stability, heavier if the objective is adductor strength.

Instruction

Lie supine on the carriage in a neutral pelvis position with the feet in the straps. Be sure the legs are straight on a diagonal line and the hips are externally rotated (see photo *a*). Inhale to open the legs into hip abduction (see photo *b*) then exhale to pull the legs into hip adduction and return to the starting position.

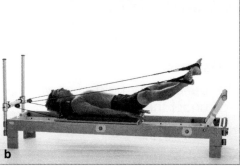

Progression

The progression for this exercise is the same as for hip extension (p. 109).

Technique Tips

1. Imagine dragging the heels through water or even mud to create internal resistance.
2. There is a tendency for the hamstrings to overpower the adductors, resulting in the legs dropping toward the floor as they are pulled in. Strive to keep the feet moving parallel to the floor as the legs open and close.
3. Keep the pelvis stable and in a neutral position throughout.

ADDUCTOR STRETCH

Primary Muscles Involved

Hip adductors

Objectives

Increased flexibility of the adductors and improved hip mobility

Indications

Tight adductors or restricted hip mobility

Precautions or Contraindications

None

Resistance

Same as for the hip work series

Instruction

After the patient has completed the hip work series on the reformer, stand inside the well, blocking the movement of the carriage with one leg and supporting the patient's legs with your hands (see photo). Have the patient take a few deep breaths and release all tension from the body, as he is supported by the carriage, straps, and instructor.

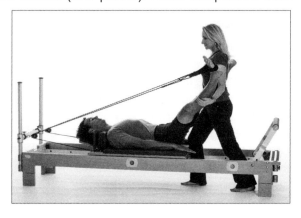

Variations

The patient can hold his own legs under the thighs.

Technique Tips

1. Make sure the pelvis is still in a neutral position.

2. The legs should drop into your hands, making it a passive stretch.
3. To come out of the stretch, first passively return the patient's legs to the midline, then step out of the well and begin the next stretch.

HAMSTRING STRETCH

Primary Muscles Involved

Hamstrings

Objectives

Increased hamstring flexibility

Indications

This provides a great way to do a manual hamstring stretch in an instructor-friendly position. It is safe for patients with low back pain, even of discogenic origin because the spine is supported and does not go into flexion. This stretch can also be done without manual assist.

Precautions or Contraindications

Acute sciatica

Resistance

Same as for the hip work series

Instruction

After the patient has completed the hip work series on the reformer, stand with one foot inside the well, blocking the movement of the carriage. Remove the strap from one foot and have the patient place that foot on the foot bar. The patient

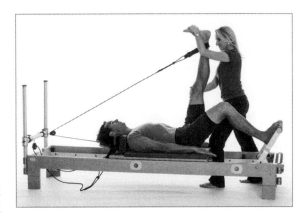

then extends the leg that is still in the strap (see photo). For an increased stretch, the patient can bend the knee of the supporting leg, which causes the rope to pull the opposite leg into more hip flexion. You can facilitate knee extension and ankle dorsiflexion, as well as ensure safety, from this position. The patient takes a few deep breaths in this position. To switch sides, first remove the patient's foot from the strap and place it on the foot bar, then follow the instructions again.

Variations

To favor the stretch toward the lateral hamstrings, slightly invert the foot and gently pull the leg toward the midline (carefully, as this can aggravate sciatica). To incline toward the medial hamstrings, evert the foot and gently pull the leg outward.

Technique Tips

1. The hip of the stretching leg should remain down on the carriage. Do not let it lift up.
2. Encourage the patient to let the leg relax and be supported by the rope.
3. Make sure the foot of the nonstretching leg maintains contact with the foot bar at all times.

SEATED BICEPS

Primary Muscles Involved

Biceps

Objectives

Biceps strength, scapular stabilization, and trunk stabilization

Indications

This is a great way to strengthen both the long head and short head of the biceps in a functional position. This exercise forces us to use the trunk muscles to keep us upright, and it forces the scapular stabilizers to keep the scapulae in the correct position. It is a good exercise for cervical patients as the neck is relaxed.

Precautions or Contraindications

None

Resistance

Light to medium

Instruction

Sit on the edge of the reformer closest to the foot bar, but facing away from it, with the hands holding the straps or handles, and the legs straight and placed in between the shoulder rests. This is known as the long sit position. Straighten the arms and lift to shoulder height, palms facing up. Set the scapulae by drawing the shoulder blades down and back (see photo a). Exhale and bend the elbows as far as possible without losing upright alignment, keeping the upper arms at the same level (see photo b). Inhale to return to the starting position.

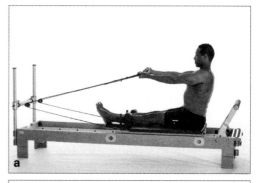

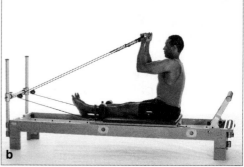

Variations

1. If the long sit position is not tolerated, the exercise can performed with bent knees (see photo *c*), sitting on a small box (see photo *d*), or in cross-legged position (see photo *e*).

2. To incorporate more abdominal work, this exercise can be performed leaning back with the lumbar spine in a deep *C*-curve. Start by drawing the abdominals in and rolling back into a posterior pelvic tilt. Hold the position that is most challenging to maintain and perform the biceps curls (see photo *f*).

Progression

To further challenge trunk stability, perform the exercise in a kneeling position as shown in the modified rows progression (see photo *c*, page 127). Lean back until there is tension in the straps and engage the abdominals by posteriorly tilting the pelvis.

Technique Tips

1. Keep the upper arms at shoulder height by imagining that they are resting on a platform throughout the exercise.

2. Straighten the arms completely on each repetition.

3. In the seated version, keep the trunk upright and make the body as tall as possible. Avoid leaning back.

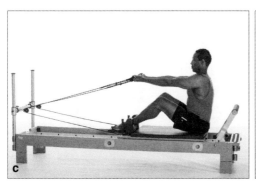
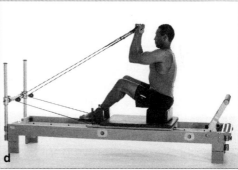
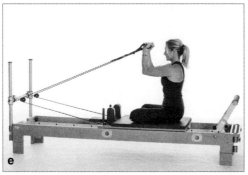
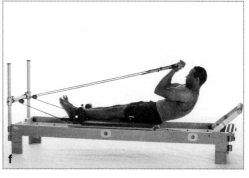

RHOMBOIDS 1

*A variation of an original exercise taught by Rael Isacowitz in the BASI Comprehensive Program (Isacowitz 2018).

Primary Muscles Involved

Rhomboids and posterior deltoids

Objectives

Shoulder abductor strength, scapular adductor strength, scapular stabilization, and trunk stabilization

Indications

This is a great exercise for general strength and function of the shoulder. I like it for both shoulder and cervical spine patients as it challenges scapular stabilization in a functional, yet generally pain free position. Protracted, rounded shoulders are a common postural problem, so isolation of scapular adduction in this exercise is an excellent way to counteract this.

Precautions or Contraindications

Early post-op rotator cuff repair

Resistance

Light

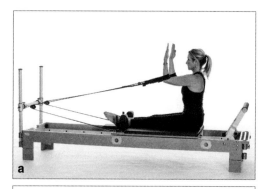

Instruction

Sit on the edge of the reformer closest to the foot bar but facing away from it, with the legs straight and the feet placed in between the shoulder rests. Reach through the straps and place them on the forearms, just below the elbows. The arms should be at shoulder height with the elbows bent to 90 degrees and the palms facing the head (see photo *a*). Exhale to horizontally abduct the shoulders, opening the arms out to the sides but keeping them at shoulder height and holding the 90 degree angle (see photo *b*). Inhale and hold. Exhale to adduct the scapulae (see photo *c*). Inhale to release the scapular adduction; then exhale and return the arms to the starting position.

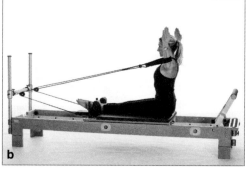

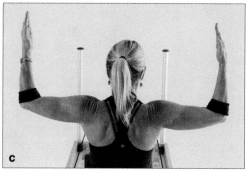

Variations

1. If the long sit position is not tolerated, the exercise can be performed with bent knees, sitting on a small box in a cross-legged position (see seated biceps variations photos *c*, *d*, and *e*, page 117).
2. For clients without adequate scapular stability and control, the scapular adduction isolation portion of the exercise can be omitted.

Progression

To further challenge trunk stability, perform the exercise in a kneeling position.

Technique Tips

1. Keep the upper arms parallel to the floor and the hands facing the head throughout the movement.
2. Maintain the "goalpost" (90 degrees of shoulder and elbow flexion) position of the arms throughout the movement.
3. The shoulders should be in slight external rotation.
4. Do not thrust the ribs forward when adducting the scapulae.
5. Keep the upper trapezius relaxed so the shoulders do not elevate.

RHOMBOIDS 2

*A variation of an original exercise taught by Rael Isacowitz in the BASI Mentor Program (Isacowitz 2018).

Primary Muscles Involved

Rhomboids and posterior deltoid

Objectives

Scapular stabilization, shoulder abductor strength, scapular adductor strength, improved posture, and trunk stabilization

Indications

The indications for this exercise are the same as for rhomboids 1 (p. 118).

Precautions or Contraindications

Early post-op rotator cuff repair

Resistance

Light

Instruction

Sit on the edge of the carriage closest to the foot bar but facing away from it with the legs threaded through the shoulder rests (ankles can be crossed). Hold the handles with the palms facing down and the arms lifted to shoulder height. Set the core muscles, lengthen the spine, and draw the shoulder blades down the back (see photo *a*). Exhale to pull the arms back, bending the elbows to a 90 degree angle at shoulder height (see photo *b*), and then inhale and hold. Exhale and draw the shoulder blades together without moving the arms, inhale as the shoulder blades are released, and then exhale and return to the starting position.

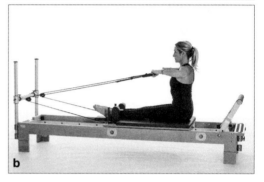

Variations

If the long sit position is not tolerated, this exercise can be performed with bent knees, sitting on a small box, or in a cross-legged position (see seated biceps variations photos *c*, *d*, and *e*, p. 117).

Progression

1. To further challenge trunk stability, perform the exercise in a kneeling position.
2. Goalpost rotator cuff (p. 120).

Technique Tips

1. Make sure the elbows remain at shoulder height throughout the exercise.
2. Keep the wrists in a neutral position.
3. Do not thrust the ribs forward when adducting the scapulae.
4. Keep the upper trapezius and levator scapulae relaxed so the shoulders do not elevate.

GOALPOST ROTATOR CUFF

*A variation of an original exercise taught by Rael Isacowitz in the BASI Powerhouse of the Upper Girdle Workshop (Isacowitz 2013).

Primary Muscles Involved

Rhomboids, posterior deltoid, and posterior rotator cuff

Objectives

Scapular stabilization, shoulder abductor strength, scapular adductor strength, rotator cuff strength and control, improved posture, and trunk stabilization

Indications

This is a very challenging shoulder exercise with the same benefits as rhomboids 1 and rhomboids 2, plus rotator cuff strengthening. It is great for athletes whose sport or position involves throwing or arm swinging (such as tennis and volleyball) as well as for swimmers as it challenges rotator cuff control in a vulnerable, yet functional position.

Precautions or Contraindications

Rotator cuff tear, early post-op rotator cuff repair, or painful tendinopathy

Resistance

Light

Instruction

This exercise is a progression of rhomboids 2, thus the set-up and beginning are the same; see photo *a*, page 119. From the point in rhomboids 2 where the arms are pulled back and the scapulae are adducted, exhale to externally rotate the shoulders to bring the arms to a goalpost position (see photo *a*). Inhale to internally rotate the shoulders back to the previous position, then exhale as the scapular adduction is released (see photo *b*), and finally inhale to bring the arms forward to the starting position.

Variations

If the long sit position is not tolerated, the exercise can be performed with knees bent, sitting on a small box, in cross-legged position, or sitting on the long box (see modified rows photo *a*, p. 127).

Progression

To further challenge trunk stability, perform the exercise in a kneeling position.

Technique Tips

In addition to the tips for rhomboids 2 (p. 119), keep the scapulae adducted as the shoulders externally and internally rotate. Each repetition of the exercise should be six distinct steps:

1. Shoulder horizontal abduction and elbow flexion
2. Scapular adduction
3. Shoulder external rotation

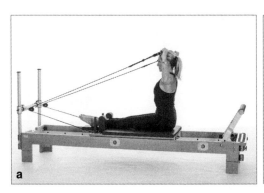
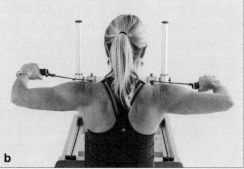

4. Shoulder internal rotation
5. Scapular abduction
6. Shoulder horizontal adduction and elbow extension

BILATERAL EXTERNAL ROTATION

*A variation of an original exercise taught by Rael Isacowitz in the BASI Powerhouse of the Upper Girdle Workshop (Isacowitz 2013).

Primary Muscles Involved

Posterior rotator cuff, middle trapezius and rhomboids

Objectives

Rotator cuff strength and control, scapular adductor strength, scapular stabilization, improved posture, and shoulder external rotation mobility

Indications

This is another great exercise to increase shoulder strength and function and scapular stabilization, as well as to improve posture as it encourages opening across the chest as opposed to rounding the back and shoulders forward. It is quite easy to perform, making it appropriate for even very weak or elderly clients. The comfortable, pain-free position of the arms at the sides makes it a favorite for conditions such as adhesive capsulitis (frozen shoulder) and impingement syndrome.

Precautions or Contraindications

Early post-op rotator cuff repair

Resistance

Light

Instruction

Sit on the edge of the carriage closest to the foot bar but facing away from it with the legs threaded through the shoulder rests (ankles can be crossed). Cross the ropes and hold the handles with the palms facing toward each other and the elbows bent to 90 degrees of flexion and pulled in against the torso. Set the core muscles, lengthen the spine, and spread wide across the collar bones to pull the scapulae into retraction, as opposed to rounding the back and shoulders forward (see photo a). Exhale and externally rotate the forearms out to the sides, as far as possible without moving the elbows from the body or cocking the wrists (see photo b). Inhale to return to the starting position.

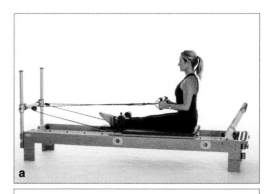

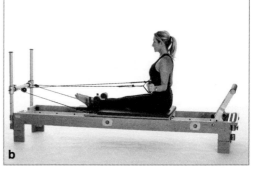

Variations

If the long sit position is not tolerated, the exercise can be performed with knees bent, sitting on a small box, in a cross-legged position, or sitting on the long box (see seated biceps variation photos c, d, and e, p. 117).

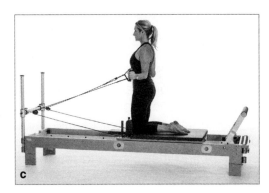

c

Progression

To further challenge trunk stability, perform the exercise in a kneeling position (see photo c).

Technique Tips

1. Keep the elbows squeezing into the waist.
2. Move the forearms parallel to the floor and keep the wrists in a neutral position throughout the exercise.
3. Palpation at the inferior angles of the scapulae with a downward and inward pull can help to activate the middle and lower trapezius.
4. Do not thrust the ribs forward when adducting the scapulae.
5. Keep the upper trapezius relaxed so the shoulders do not elevate.

CHEST EXPANSION WIDE

*A variation of an original exercise taught by Rael Isacowitz in the BASI Mentor Program (Isacowitz 2018).

Primary Muscles Involved

Posterior deltoids, middle trapezius, and rhomboids

Objectives

Shoulder horizontal abduction strength, scapular adductor strength, scapular stabilization, and improved posture

Indications

This is primarily a postural exercise as it opens the chest and counteracts rounded shoulder posture. It is wonderful for people who sit at a computer for hours.

Precautions or Contraindications

None

Resistance

Light

Instruction

Sit on the edge of the carriage closest to the foot bar but facing away from it with the legs threaded through the shoulder rests (ankles can be crossed). Cross the ropes and hold the handles with the palms facing toward each other and the arms lifted to shoulder height (see photo *a*). Set the core muscles, lengthen the spine, and spread wide across the collar bones to pull the scapulae into retraction. Exhale and open the arms out to the sides (see photo *b*) and then inhale to return to the starting position.

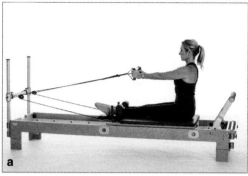

Variations

If the long sit position is not tolerated, the exercise can be performed with knees bent, sitting on a small box, in cross-legged position, or sitting on the long box (see modified rows photo *a*, p. 127).

Progression

To further challenge trunk stability, perform the exercise in a kneeling position. This will also increase the

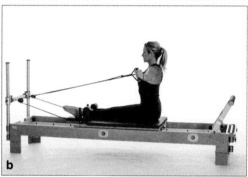

challenge of the scapular depressors as the angle of resistance in this position elicits activation of the upper trapezius.

Technique Tips

1. Move the arms parallel to the floor and keep the wrists neutral throughout the exercise.
2. Manual cueing via palpation at the inferior angles of the scapulae with a downward and inward pull can help to activate the middle and lower trapezius.
3. Do not thrust the ribs forward when adducting the scapulae.
4. Keep the upper trapezius relaxed so the shoulders do not elevate.
5. Keep the arms fully extended but the elbows soft—not hyperextended and not overly bent.
6. The shoulders should be in slight external rotation.
7. If in the kneeling position, maintain an upright position and slightly posteriorly tilt the pelvis to elicit engagement of the abdominals and a stretch of the hip flexors.

HUG A TREE

Primary Muscles Involved

Pectoralis major and minor

Objectives

Shoulder horizontal adduction strength and control, scapular stabilization, and improved posture

Indications

Often working the pecs can result in rounded shoulders, so the ability to avoid this when pulling into horizontal adduction, as instructed in this exercise, is very valuable.

Precautions or Contraindications

None

Resistance

Light to medium

Instruction

Sit upright on the carriage facing the foot bar, with the hips against the shoulder rests and the legs reaching directly forward. Hold the handles or straps and reach the arms out to a *T* position with the shoulders slightly externally rotated, keeping the elbows straight but not locked and the palms facing forward (see photo *a*). Exhale to bring the arms toward each other, keeping them in line with the shoulders (see photo *b*), then inhale to open the arms and return to the starting position without moving the scapulae.

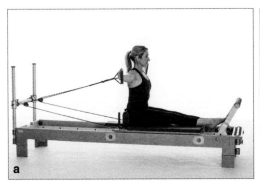
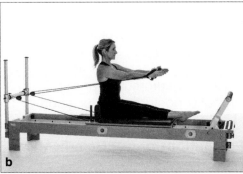

Variations

If the long sit position is not tolerated, perform the exercise with knees bent, sitting on a small pad to elevate the pelvis, in a cross-legged position, or sitting on the long box.

Progression

To further challenge trunk stability, perform the exercise in a kneeling position.

Technique Tips

1. Emphasize external rotation of the shoulders by leading the movement with the little finger.
2. Move the arms parallel to the floor.
3. Keep the upper trapezius relaxed so the shoulders do not elevate.
4. To help prevent rounding of the thoracic spine and shoulders, focus on the mid and upper back extensors.
5. Elongate the arms out to the sides without hyperextending the elbows.
6. If in the kneeling position, maintain an upright position and slightly posteriorly tilt the pelvis to elicit engagement of the abdominals and a stretch of the hip flexors.

MODIFIED ROWS

Primary Muscles Involved

Latissimus dorsi, middle trapezius, and rhomboids

Objectives

Upper and middle back strength, improved posture, and scapular stabilization

Indications

This exercise is a favorite for my elderly patients, as the position is comfortable and safe for them, and the movement is beneficial yet easy to execute. Yet it is also very effective for anyone who needs strengthening of the upper back muscles, neuromuscular retraining of the scapular stabilizers, or decreased kyphotic posture. The position of the arms makes it appropriate for most shoulder injuries, including adhesive capsulitis and impingement syndrome.

Precautions or Contraindications

None

Resistance

Medium to heavy

Instruction

Sit on the long box facing away from the foot bar with the feet on the headrest and the knees squeezing together. Cross the ropes and hold the handles with the palms facing each other and the arms extended (see photo a). Sit up tall with the abdominals engaged and the shoulder blades drawing toward the back pockets; then exhale as the arms pull backwards and the elbows reach past the torso. The hands stay at waist level (see photo b). Inhale to return to the starting position.

Progression

Perform the exercise in a kneeling position with the feet hooked over the back edge of the carriage (see photo c). The heavy springs will pull the torso forward and down toward the well, so use caution. This version takes a great deal of core control and balance to stabilize the trunk.

Technique Tips

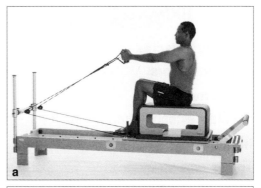
a

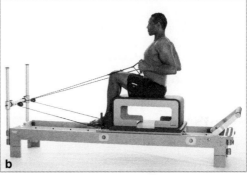
b

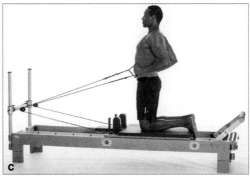
c

1. Consciously pull the arms back behind the torso and resist the pull of the ropes when returning the arms forward, rather than swinging the arms back and forth.

2. Keep the arms close to the torso throughout the exercise.

3. Palpation at the inferior angles of the scapulae with a downward and inward pull can help to activate the middle and lower trapezius as instructed in activation of the lower trapezius in chapter 4, p. 43.

4. Do not thrust the ribs forward when adducting the scapulae.

5. Keep the neck relaxed and the shoulders away from the ears.

6. Use the abdominals and back extensors to ensure an upright posture. Elongate through the crown of the head to grow as tall as possible.

7. If in the kneeling position, maintain an upright position and slightly posteriorly tilt the pelvis to elicit engagement of the abdominals and a stretch through the hip flexors.

CHEST EXPANSION

Primary Muscles Involved

Latissimus dorsi

Objectives

Shoulder extensor strength, trunk stabilization, core control, and improved posture

Indications

This is one of my favorite exercises to improve posture! It encourages activation of the scapular stabilizers as well as opening of the shoulders, while the neck is relaxed. The exercise also challenges upright trunk posture and core control.

Precautions or Contraindications

The kneeling position can be difficult for people with knee pain or those who lack core control.

Resistance

Light

Instruction

Kneel on the reformer facing away from the foot bar with the knees against the shoulder rests, holding the ropes with the palms facing the sides of the body. The arms should be slightly forward of the trunk (see photo *a*). Inhale to set the core and spread wide across the collar bones drawing the shoulder blades down and back. Exhale and pull the arms back as far as possible without losing the upright alignment of the trunk (see photo *b*), then inhale to return to the starting position.

Variations

1. For those who cannot tolerate the kneeling position or do not have enough core stability to perform this exercise safely, the exercise can be performed sitting on the long box (as in modified rows photos *a* and *b*, p.127) or in the long sit position.

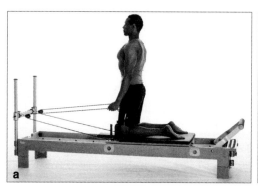 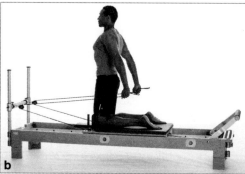

2. To improve cervical spine mobility and teach dissociation of the head from the trunk, add rotation of the head. When the ropes are pulled back, hold the position and rotate the head slowly to the left, to the right, and back to center. Return the ropes to the starting position. This is very effective for those who tend to tense the upper trapezius and levator scapulae muscles whenever an upper body exercise is executed (or even mentioned). Rotation of the head while the arms are engaged demonstrates the ability to achieve simultaneous upper back muscle activation and neck relaxation.

Technique Tips

1. If in the kneeling position, maintain an upright position and slightly posteriorly tilt the pelvis to elicit engagement of the abdominals and a stretch through the hip flexors.
2. Lengthen through the arms.
3. Consciously pull the arms back behind the torso and resist the pull of the ropes when returning the arms forward, rather than swinging the arms back and forth.

SHOULDER INTERNAL ROTATION

Primary Muscles Involved

Subscapularis

Objectives

Rotator cuff strength and control and scapular stabilization

Indications

This exercise is great for shoulder weakness due to rotator cuff tendinosis or tear, postsurgical repair, adhesive capsulitis, impingement syndrome, or labral tear. It is also good for improving or maintaining shoulder rotation range of motion.

Precautions or Contraindications

None

Resistance

Light

Instruction

Sit on the long box facing sideways on the carriage, holding one handle in the arm closest to the ropes with the elbow at 90 degrees of flexion and pressing into the torso, and with the wrist in a neutral position. Place a small rolled towel or ball between the elbow and the torso (see photo a). Engage the abdominals, elongate the spine, and draw the shoulder blade toward the opposite back pocket. Exhale to internally rotate the shoulder (see photo b) and inhale while returning to the starting position.

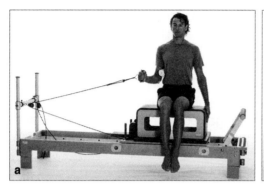 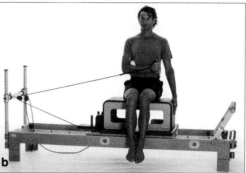

Progression

To challenge trunk stability, perform the exercise in a kneeling position.

Technique Tips

1. Keep the scapular stabilizing muscles engaged throughout by drawing the shoulder blade down and back.
2. Keep the wrist in a neutral position.

SHOULDER EXTERNAL ROTATION

Primary Muscles Involved

Supraspinatus, infraspinatus, and teres minor

Objectives

Rotator cuff strength and control, shoulder rotation range of motion, and scapular stabilization

Indications

The indications for this exercise are the same as for shoulder internal rotation (p. 129).

Precautions or Contraindications

Early post-op rotator cuff repair

Resistance

Extra light. It may be necessary to move the carriage gear bar farther away from the foot bar to decrease the resistance.

Instruction

Sit on the long box facing sideways on the carriage, holding one handle in the arm closest to the foot bar with the elbow at 90 degrees of flexion and pressing into the torso, and the wrist in a neutral position. Place a small rolled towel or ball between the elbow and the torso (see photo *a*). Engage the abdominals, elongate the spine, and draw the shoulder blade toward the opposite back pocket. Exhale to externally rotate the shoulder (see photo *b*), then inhale to return to the starting position.

Progression

Perform the exercise in a kneeling position to challenge trunk stabilization.

Technique Tips

The tips for this exercise are the same as for shoulder internal rotation (p. 129).

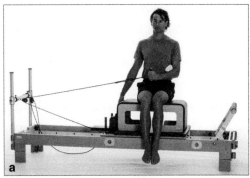

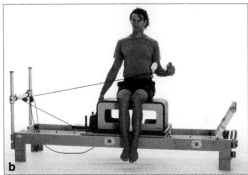

SHOULDER DIAGONAL PULL (MODIFIED CROSS ARM PULL)

Primary Muscles Involved

Rotator cuff muscles, shoulder flexors, and shoulder abductors

Objectives

Functional shoulder strength and control, scapular stabilization, rotator cuff strength, and shoulder ROM

Indications

This exercise requires effective proprioceptive communication between the muscles and the joints, resulting in a balance of mobility and stability and producing a functional movement. It is an adaptation of cross arm pull, which is taught in the BASI comprehensive program. The movement in this exercise follows what is known as the PNF D2 pattern of the shoulder. Proprioceptive neuromuscular facilitation (PNF) is a concept widely used in rehabilitation to improve the neuromuscular system's effectiveness in coordinating movement. The facilitation incorporates mass movement patterns that are diagonal and spiral in nature and often cross the midline of the body. Upper extremity patterns are used to treat dysfunction caused by muscular weakness, incoordination, and joint restrictions. The arm patterns are also used to exercise the trunk. (Adler, Beckers, and Buck 1993). Although the resistance in this exercise is not manual as in a true PNF technique, the spring resistance provided by the reformer in the D2 pattern makes it a wonderful exercise because it challenges the scapular and trunk stabilizers in a functional pattern, while at the same time strengthening the more distal muscles of the arm and challenging coordination.

Precautions or Contraindications

Acute shoulder impingement syndrome, early post-op rotator cuff repair, or pain with overhead motion

Resistance

Extra light

Instruction

Sit sideways on the long box holding one handle in the opposite hand with the arm reaching across the body to the opposite hip; the shoulder is internally rotated, and the palm is facing the body (see photo a). Exhale to pull the arm across the body in a diagonal pattern, gradually externally rotating

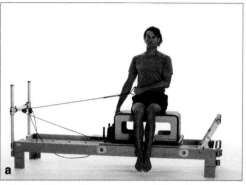

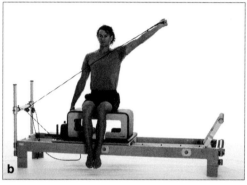

the shoulder and supinating the forearm as the arm elevates (see photo b). Inhale and return to the starting position, gradually internally rotating the shoulder on the way down.

Progression

To challenge trunk stability and thus increase the overall PNF required to achieve the movement, perform the exercise in a kneeling position.

Technique Tips

1. The movement across the body should be in a smooth diagonal pattern.
2. When full shoulder elevation is reached, the shoulder should be in maximal external rotation and the thumb facing backwards.

ARMS OVERHEAD

Primary Muscles Involved

Deltoids

Objectives

Shoulder abductor strength, scapular stabilization, and improved scapulohumeral rhythm

Indications

This is a wonderful exercise for anyone recovering from a shoulder injury and going back to a sport, as it retrains proper functioning of scapulohumeral rhythm. It is very challenging to maintain scapular and trunk stabilization as one arm is pulling against the resistance of the spring while the other is not.

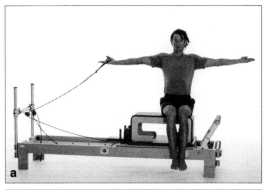

Precautions or Contraindications

Shoulder impingement syndrome, rotator cuff tendinitis or tear, labral tear, or pain with overhead motion

Resistance

Extra light

Instruction

Sit sideways close to the foot bar on the long box and hold one handle in the hand closest to the ropes with the arms in a *T* position with the palms

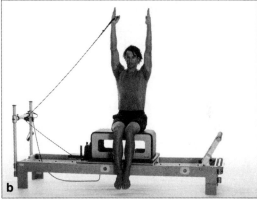

facing up (see photo *a*). Exhale and lift both arms overhead (see photo *b*), then inhale to lower the arms to the starting position.

Progression

To challenge trunk stability and make the exercise both more functional and more difficult, perform in a kneeling position with the legs shoulder-width apart and the outer leg at the front edge of the carriage.

Technique Tips

1. Counteract upper trapezius overactivity by maintaining scapular depression throughout.
2. Both arms should lift and lower symmetrically and look as if they are working against equal resistance.
3. Keep the trunk upright and centered, avoiding lateral flexion.

KNEELING ARM CIRCLES

Primary Muscles Involved

Deltoids

Objectives

Shoulder flexor strength and scapular and trunk stabilization

Indications

Because this exercise goes into the overhead position, it is very challenging for shoulder strength and scapular stability. It also helps increase or maintain shoulder elevation range of motion. It is especially useful for shoulder rehabilitation of overhead sport athletes such as swimmers, volleyball players, tennis players, and water polo players. It also challenges core control and trunk stabilization. For nonathletes, it is still very useful since we all need to be able to reach and lift overhead with a stable scapula.

Precautions or Contraindications

Shoulder impingement syndrome, rotator cuff tendinitis or tear, early to mid-stage status post– rotator cuff repair, or pain with overhead motion

Resistance

Light

Instruction

Kneel on the carriage facing the foot bar with feet pressed against the shoulder rests, hands in the straps or handles, and arms by the sides of the body with the palms facing forward (see photo *a*). Continue with up circles or down circles as explained next.

Up Circles

Exhale as the arms lift into shoulder flexion (see photo *b*). When the arms reach maximum elevation (see photo *c*), rotate the palms to face forward and inhale as the arms lower to a *T* position, (see photo *d*) and then return to the starting position.

Down Circles

This exercise is the same as up circles but in reverse order. Start in the same position and then exhale to raise arms out to a *T* position and continue up until they are overhead. At maximum elevation rotate the palms to the back, then inhale as the arms are lowered to the starting position with the palms facing up.

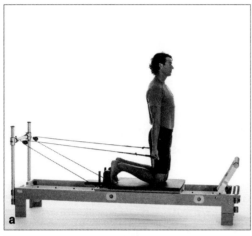
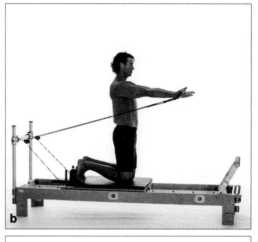
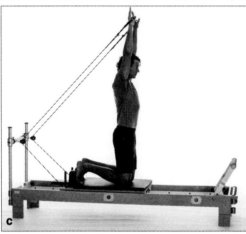
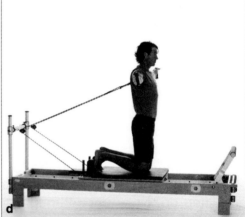

Variations

For a weaker client with inadequate trunk stabilization or to focus only on shoulder ROM, the exercise can be performed from a straddle sit position on the long box.

Technique Tips

1. Keep the movement smooth as in supine arm circles on p. 99, presented earlier in this chapter.
2. Do not let the hands go behind the torso.
3. Keep the core engaged and maintain the upright position of the trunk.
4. Keep the scapulae depressed so the shoulders do not rise up toward the ears as the arms are elevated.

KNEELING BICEPS

*A variation of an original exercise taught by Rael Isacowitz in the BASI Mentor Program (Isacowitz 2018).

Primary Muscles Involved

Biceps

Objectives

Elbow flexor strength, scapular adductor strength, shoulder flexor stretch, scapular and trunk stabilization, and improved posture

Indications

This exercise gives us an excellent alternative position in which to work the biceps—one that counteracts the tendency to round the shoulders forward and use the pecs. With the arms behind the back, the chest is open and the scapular adductors are working. This position and the direction of resistance also challenge scapular and trunk stabilization.

Precautions or Contraindications

None

Resistance

Medium

Instruction

Kneel on the carriage facing the foot bar with the feet pressed against the shoulder rests. Hold the handles or straps with the arms reaching backwards and lifted up. Draw back through the elbows as the collar bones lift (see photo a). Exhale to bend the elbows (see photo b), and inhale to return to the starting position.

Variations

For a weaker client with inadequate trunk stabilization, the exercise can be performed from a straddle sit position on the long box.

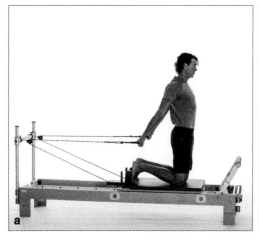
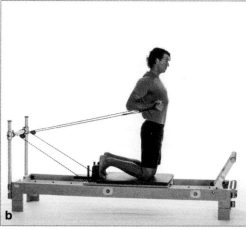

Technique Tips

1. Keep the elbows and upper arms still and parallel to each other.
2. Spread wide across the collar bones and keep the scapular adductors engaged to keep the shoulder heads from falling or rounding forward.
3. Avoid thrusting the ribs forward.

QUADRUPED ABS (MODIFIED KNEE STRETCH)

Primary Muscles Involved

Abdominals

Objectives

Lumbo-pelvic stabilization, scapular stabilization, and hip and knee extensor strength and control

Indications

This exercise is categorized in BASI Pilates as full-body integration. Exercises in this category rely on integration of the whole body for performance, rather than on a single region. Full-body integration exercises are closed chain, which makes them very functional and thus crucial in injury rehab. Classically, this exercise is called knee stretch, and it has both a round back and a flat back version. For both practical and documentation purposes, I prefer this version and the name quadruped abs or modified knee stretch. It is one of my favorite exercises for all low back pain patients because it can easily be modified based on the pathology, and it works the rectus abdominis eccentrically. It is also a great exercise for scapular stabilization and hip dissociation.

Precautions or Contraindications

Patients with lumbar disk pathology or osteoporosis should avoid the round back version, and those with spondylolisthesis or stenosis should avoid the flat back position. If the position causes knee pain, a pad placed underneath the knees will alleviate this.

Resistance

Extra light

Instruction

Get in a quadruped position on the reformer with the foot bar down. The hands are on the base of the reformer and the knees are directly under the hips. Shift the body and the carriage back a few inches (several centimeters), so the shoulders are in approximately 120 degrees of flexion rather than directly over the hands. This will pre-tension the springs (see photo *a*). Inhale to set the core then extend at the hips to push the carriage back, keeping the shoulders and trunk stable (see photo *b*), then exhale to return to the starting position.

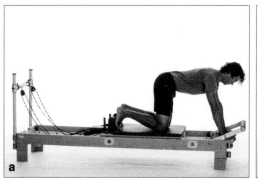 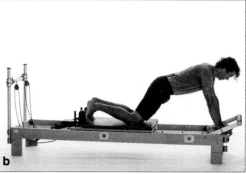

Variations

For patients with disk pathologies or osteoporosis, the lumbar spine should be in a neutral position or even slight extension (flat back position). For patients with stenosis or spondylolisthesis, the lumbar spine should remain in flexion throughout the exercise (round back position).

Progression

Perform the exercise with no springs.

Technique Tips

1. Think of the abdominals pulling the carriage in, not the arms.
2. Draw the shoulder blades down and back into the back pockets.
3. Hinge only at the hips; nothing else should move.

REVERSE QUADRUPED ABS

*A variation of an original exercise taught by Rael Isacowitz in the BASI Comprehensive Program (Isacowitz 2018).

Primary Muscles Involved

Abdominals and hip flexors

Objectives

Lumbo-pelvic stabilization, scapular stabilization, and hip flexor strength and control

Indications

The indications for this exercise are the same as for quadruped abs (p. 137), except that this version emphasizes concentric abdominal work.

Precautions or Contraindications

Hip flexor injuries in addition to the precautions for quadruped abs (p. 137)

Resistance

Light

Instruction

Get in a quadruped position on the reformer facing away from the foot bar. Knees are pressed against the shoulder rests and the hands are on the rails slightly forward of the shoulders with slight tension on the springs. Round the lower back, pulling into a deep C-curve and setting the core (see photo a). Exhale to draw the knees in toward the hands, pulling in to an even deeper C-curve (see photo b). Inhale to return the carriage back to the starting position, keeping the trunk in flexion.

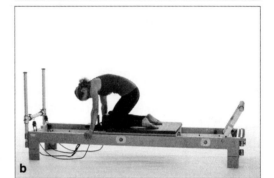

Variations

For patients with disk pathology or osteoporosis, the spine should be kept in a neutral position (flat back) instead of in a round-back position throughout the exercise. However, this puts the abdominals at a mechanical disadvantage, giving more load to the hip flexors and therefore possibly causing more stress on the lower back.

Technique Tips

1. Use the abdominals to pull the carriage in, not the arms or the hip flexors.
2. Keep the shoulder blades drawn down and back.
3. Maintain the deep C-curve throughout the exercise (if appropriate).

QUADRUPED TRICEPS KICKBACK

Primary Muscles Involved

Triceps

Objectives

Triceps strength and tone, scapular stabilization, and core stabilization

Indications

This is a wonderful exercise because in addition to strengthening the triceps, trunk and scapular stabilization are challenged. To achieve the proper position of the scapula, the serratus anterior, lower trapezius, and latissimus dorsi of the supporting arm must be activated.

Precautions or Contraindications

If the position causes knee pain, a pad placed underneath the knees should alleviate this.

Resistance

Light to Medium

Instruction

Get in a quadruped position on the carriage facing away from the foot bar with the knees directly under the hips and the spine in a neutral position. Place one hand on the headrest directly under the shoulder. Press down into the headrest while drawing the shoulder blade toward the pelvis to set the scapular stabilizers. Hold the handle with the opposite hand facing the body and then lift that arm so it is level with the torso; the elbow is bent and hugging the rib cage (see photo *a*). Exhale and straighten the elbow, bringing the arm into full extension while keeping the upper arm still (see photo *b*), then inhale to bend the elbow and return to the starting position.

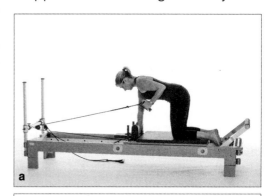

Progression

To further challenge trunk stability, perform the exercise with the opposite leg extended (see photo *c*).

Technique Tips

1. Avoid a winging scapula of the supporting side by pressing down into the palm to encourage activation of the serratus anterior, lower trapezius, and latissimus dorsi.

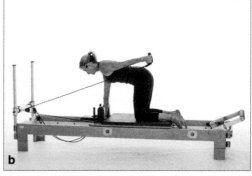

2. Keep the core muscles engaged but the neck muscles relaxed.

3. Keep the shoulder of the moving arm pulled back and up, not allowing it to dip forward.

4. In the advanced version, hold the extended leg at hip height without changing the position of the pelvis and make the leg as long as possible.

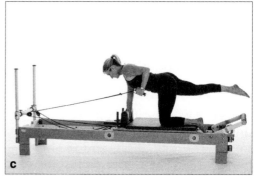

UP STRETCH 1

Primary Muscles Involved

Abdominals and back extensors

Objectives

Shoulder and trunk stabilization; core strength; and improved flexibility of hamstrings, calves, and shoulder

Indications

Shoulder stability and mobility are increased in this closed-chain exercise that demands cocontraction of the shoulder musculature, as well as the abdominals and back extensors. As with other full body integration exercises, using less resistance increases the level of difficulty by challenging core strength and stabilization. The body pivots around the shoulder joint to minimize stress on the shoulders while challenging control. Scapular adduction and depression are challenged to avoid elevation and protraction.

Precautions or Contraindications

Weak core or poor core control, shoulder impingement syndrome, early post-op rotator cuff or labral repair, as well as lumbar disk pathologies if the patient is unable to avoid lumbar flexion in the up stretch position due to tight hamstrings or lack of hip mobility

Resistance

Light to medium

Instruction

Stand on the carriage with the hands on the foot bar, arms straight and shoulder-width apart, heels halfway up the shoulder rests. The head should be between the arms, the pelvis lifted toward the ceiling, and the back flat (see photo *a*). Inhale to hinge at the hip joint to push the carriage slightly back (see photo *b*). Stabilize with the trunk and shoulders. Exhale as the abdominals draw in and pull the carriage back toward the stopper, returning to the starting position.

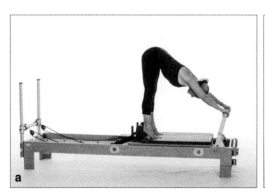
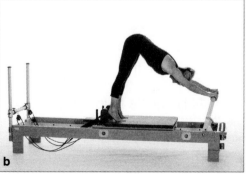

Variations

Instead of lifting the heels halfway up the shoulder rests, keep the feet flat on the carriage. This version, called elephant, increases the hamstring and calf stretch and gives an increased feeling of stability.

Progression

Up stretch 2 (p. 142) and long stretch (p. 143)

Technique Tips

1. Keep the head aligned with the spine.
2. Keep the tailbone reaching upward.
3. Maintain a pyramid shape with the body, drawing the chest toward the thighs to keep a straight back.
4. Keep the trunk as stable as possible in a neutral position.
5. Swing the legs back and forth from the hip joints like a pendulum.
6. Emphasize the inward phase of the motion.
7. Avoid scapular elevation by pulling the shoulders down toward the hips.

UP STRETCH 2

Primary Muscles Involved

Abdominals and back extensors

Objectives

Shoulder and trunk stabilization; core strength; and improved flexibility of hamstrings, calves, and shoulder

Indications

The indications for this exercise are the same as for up stretch 1 (p. 141).

Precautions or Contraindications

Same as for up stretch 1 (p. 141)

Resistance

Light

Instruction

The setup for this exercise is the same as for up stretch 1 (see photo *a*, p. 141). Inhale to lower the body as the legs push the carriage back, keeping the arms still and pivoting around the shoulder and hip joints until a plank position is reached (see photo). Exhale to lift the pelvis

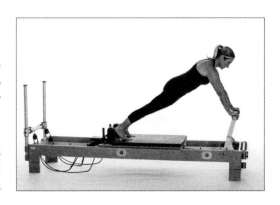

to the ceiling and pull the carriage back in to the stopper, again pivoting at the shoulder and hip joints.

Progression

Long stretch (p. 143), up stretch 3 (p. 144)

Technique Tips

The tips for this exercise are the same as for up stretch 1 (p. 141).

LONG STRETCH

Primary Muscles Involved

Abdominals and scapular stabilizers

Objectives

Shoulder and trunk stabilization, core strength, and shoulder flexor strength

Indications

The indications for this exercise are the same as for up stretch 1 (p.141), but this exercise requires even more abdominal strength, core control, and stabilization.

Precautions or Contraindications

Weak core or poor core control, shoulder impingement syndrome, or early post-op rotator cuff or labral repair

Resistance

Light

Instruction

Start in the up stretch 1 position (photo a, p. 141). Lower the body to a plank position by pivoting around the shoulder and hip joints as in up stretch 2 (see photo, p. 142). Inhale to glide the body forward toward the foot bar until the carriage reaches the stopper (see photo). Exhale to push the carriage back to the starting position. While holding the plank position, continue to glide the carriage forward and back 5 to 10 times.

Progression

Up stretch 3 (p. 144)

Technique Tips

1. Tilt the pelvis slightly posteriorly to help ensure engagement of the abdominals and avoid hyperlordosis.

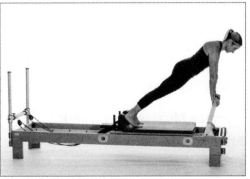

2. Keep the head aligned with the spine.
3. Spread wide across the collar bones and draw the shoulder blades down the back throughout.

UP STRETCH 3

Primary Muscles Involved

Abdominals, back extensors, and scapular stabilizers

Objectives

Shoulder and trunk stabilization; core strength; shoulder flexor strength; and improved flexibility of hamstrings, calves, and shoulder

Indications

This exercise is a combination and progression of up stretch 2 and long stretch.

Precautions or Contraindications

Weak core or poor core control, shoulder impingement syndrome, early post-op rotator cuff or labral repair, as well as lumbar disk pathologies if the patient is unable to avoid lumbar flexion in the up stretch position due to tight hamstrings or lack of hip mobility

Resistance

Light

Instruction

Start in the up stretch 1 position (see up stretch 1 photo, *a*, page 141). Inhale to lower the body to the long stretch position (see up stretch 2, photo, p 142). Glide forward until the carriage reaches the stopper (see long stretch photo, p. 143). Exhale to lift the pelvis and return to the starting position (see up stretch 1 photo *a*, page 141).

Technique Tips

1. Follow all of the tips from up stretch 1 (p. 141) and long stretch (p. 143).
2. Deeply engage the abdominals to initiate the transition from the long stretch position to the up stretch position.
3. Press the carriage firmly against the stopper when transitioning from the long stretch to the up stretch position.

DOWN STRETCH

Primary Muscles Involved

Abdominals and upper back extensors

Objectives

Trunk and scapular stabilization, shoulder extensor and upper back extensor control, and improved posture

Indications

This exercise demands a great deal of trunk stabilization, as well as scapular and pelvic control. If these are not adequate, the lumbar spine goes into hyperlordosis, resulting in excessive pressure. Using less resistance increases the level of difficulty by challenging core strength and stabilization. It is another wonderful exercise for people with thoracic kyphosis or rounded shoulders as it counteracts these postures.

Precautions or Contraindications

Spondylolisthesis, stenosis, weak core, or poor core control

Resistance

Light

Instruction

Kneel on the carriage with the feet pressing against the shoulder rests and the hands on the foot bar, shoulder-width apart with straight arms. The body in an arc shape with the pelvis pulled into a slight posterior tilt. Spread wide across the collar bones and strive for maximum thoracic extension (see photo *a*). Exhale and pivot from the shoulders to push the carriage back while maintaining the arc shape of the body (see photo *b*). Inhale and press down into the foot bar to lift the body back to the starting position. The carriage should touch the stopper and maximum thoracic extension should again be reached, without going into too much lumbar lordosis.

Technique Tips

1. Keep the abdominals engaged and the pelvis in a slight posterior tilt throughout the exercise to protect the lumbar spine.
2. Keep the back, hip, and shoulder extensors working throughout the movement, striving to maintain the body in a consistent arc shape.
3. Imagine that the body is the figurehead of a ship, with the sternum lifting the body up and over the waves.

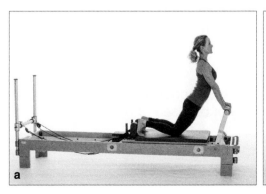
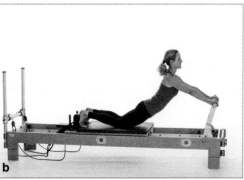

SHOULDER PUSH

*A variation of an original exercise taught by Rael Isacowitz in the BASI Master I and Master II Programs (Isacowitz 2018).

Primary Muscles Involved

Abdominals and scapular stabilizers

Objectives

Trunk and scapular stabilization, core control, and shoulder strength and control

Indications

This exercise introduces closed-chain work for the shoulders without stressing the wrists or placing the shoulder in a contraindicated position for injuries such as impingement syndrome or adhesive capsulitis. It challenges scapular and core stabilization and control in a less precarious position than in the up stretch exercises. The plank on elbows position has demonstrated muscle coactivation without external loading on the lumbar spine in electromyogram studies and is thus beneficial for stabilization and endurance training for improved athletic performance and injury prevention (Ekstrom, Donatelli, and Carp 2007). Maintaining this position on an unstable surface makes it even more challenging to the core stabilizers.

Precautions or Contraindications

Lumbar disk pathologies if the patient is unable to avoid lumbar flexion in this exercise due to tight hamstrings or lack of hip mobility, and early post-op rotator cuff repair

Resistance

Light

Instruction

Place the foot bar in the lowest position. Kneel on the carriage facing the shoulder rests and place the elbows in the middle of the carriage with the palms facing each other and pressing down into the bottom of the shoulder rests. Place one foot on the foot bar and push the carriage out (see photo a). Carefully lift the opposite foot and place it on the foot bar, achieving the plank on elbows position (see photo b). Draw the shoulder blades down and back and activate the core muscles. Exhale to lift the hips and pull the carriage back to the stopper, bringing the chest toward the thighs (see photo c). Inhale to return to the plank position.

Progression

The foot bar can be raised or the exercise can be performed with one leg lifted a few inches (several centimeters) off the foot bar (see photo d).

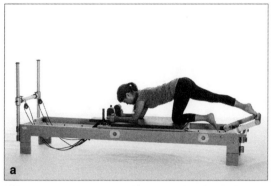 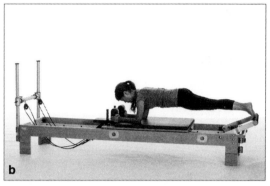

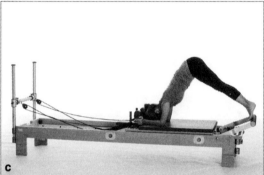 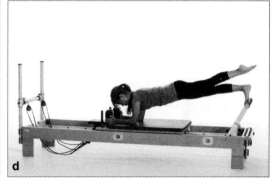

Technique Tips

1. Keep the core muscles engaged throughout.
2. Relax the head and neck, keeping the head in line with the spine.
3. Draw the elbows toward each other. They should be directly under the shoulders, not splaying out to the sides.
4. Keep the hips level with the rest of the body when in the plank position.

MODIFIED BALANCE CONTROL FRONT

Primary Muscles Involved

Abdominals and scapular stabilizers

Objectives

Trunk and scapular stabilization, core control, and shoulder strength and control

Indications

The indications are the same as for shoulder push (p. 146). This exercise removes the hip flexion component but still requires a great deal of abdominal strength, core control, and scapular stabilization.

Precautions or Contraindications

Early post-op rotator cuff repair

Resistance

Light

Instruction

The setup and starting position for this exercise are the same as for shoulder push (see photo *b*, page 147). Exhale to press the carriage a few inches (several centimeters) forward while maintaining the plank position (see photo *a*). Inhale as the carriage is pulled back in to the starting position (see photo *b*).

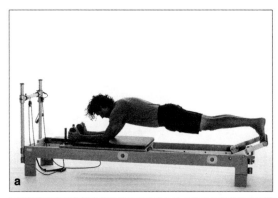

Progression

The foot bar can be raised or the exercise can be performed with one leg lifted a few inches (several centimeters) off the foot bar.

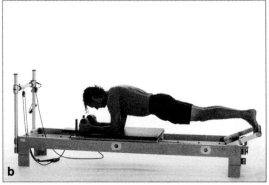

Technique Tips

The tips for this exercise are the same as for shoulder push (p. 146).

SKATING HYBRID

*A variation of an original exercise taught by Rael Isacowitz in the BASI Comprehensive Program (Isacowitz 2018).

Primary Muscles Involved

Gluteus medius and quadriceps

Objectives

Hip abductor strength, lumbo-pelvic stabilization, knee stabilization and control, and proper patellofemoral alignment

Indications

This exercise is a great one for athletes because it strengthens the hip abductors in a functional position, challenges knee stability and control, and encourages proper patellofemoral alignment. Of course, the core muscles are also working to maintain lumbo-pelvic stabilization.

Precautions or Contraindications

Non–weight-bearing status

Resistance

Medium

Instruction

Stand on the foot plate or standing platform with the right foot and place the left foot on the edge of the carriage, parallel to the right foot. Take an athletic stance by bending both knees and flexing at the hips but keeping the back straight. Keep the left kneecap aligned over the second and third toes. Hands are on the hips or behind the back (see photo *a*). Exhale to dynamically press the carriage away and straighten only the right leg (see photo *b*) and then inhale to return the carriage to the stopper slowly and with control. The left leg stabilizes while the right leg moves.

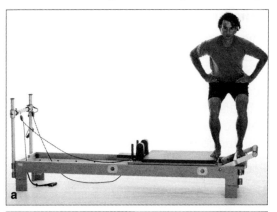

Variation

Reverse skating: Make the right leg the stabilizer as the left leg presses the carriage out (see photo *c*).

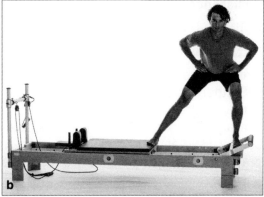

Technique Tips

1. Keep the trunk and stabilizing leg completely still as the other leg pushes the carriage out.

2. Press into the heel of the stabilizing leg.

3. This exercise should be felt in the glutes. If it is not, flex a bit more at the hips and knees.

4. Visualize a speed skater pushing off forcefully but returning with grace and control.

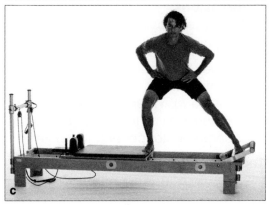

SIDE SPLITS

Primary Muscles Involved

Hip adductors

Objectives

Hip adductor strength and control and lumbo-pelvic stabilization

Indications

This exercise provides an easy way to strengthen the often weak adductors in a functional, standing position. It also provides a great stretch while maximizing hip range of motion. The pressing-out phase works the adductors eccentrically while the pulling-in phase works them concentrically. The exercise also requires coordinated activation of the abdominals, pelvic floor, and back extensors to keep the body in an upright, neutral pelvis position. Light resistance is necessary so that the abductors do not take over.

Precautions or Contraindications

Non–weight-bearing status

Resistance

Light

Instruction

Stand on the reformer with the left foot on the platform as in skating hybrid (p. 148), then place the right foot on a nonslip pad as far out as possible on the carriage. Hold the arms up in a *T* position (see photo *a*). Inhale and allow the carriage to move away from the foot bar as far as possible while maintaining control. Hold at the end of the range for a few seconds (see photo *b*). Exhale to draw the carriage back to the starting position, squeezing the thighs together until the carriage presses against the stopper.

Progressions

1. If the patient has long legs and is very strong and flexible, the foot can be placed against the shoulder rest.
2. If you have a standing platform attachment, the exercise can be performed in hip external rotation, which is a great position for dancers to train in (see photo *c*). When the carriage is out, bend the knees to a squat position without letting the carriage move (see photo *d*), then pull the carriage back in to the stopper and straighten the legs.

Technique Tips

1. Posteriorly tilt the pelvis slightly to engage the abdominals and protect the lumbar spine.
2. There is a tendency to lean forward during the movement. To counteract this keep the trunk upright, lengthening through the top of the head.

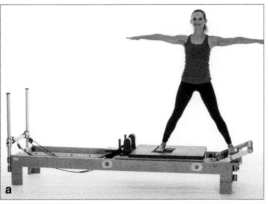
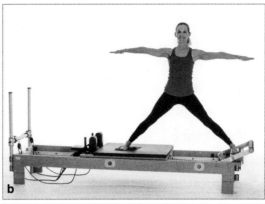
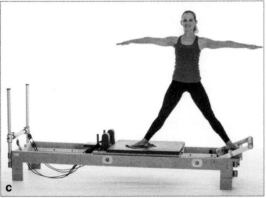
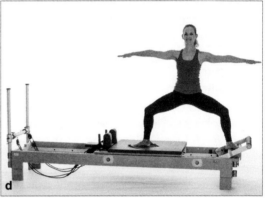

3. Keep the shoulder blades drawn down the back and the collar bones spread apart.

4. Think of lifting the body toward the ceiling and squeezing a large ball between the legs when pulling the carriage in.

TERMINAL KNEE EXTENSION

Primary Muscles Involved

Quadriceps

Objectives

Neuromuscular reeducation of the vastus medialis oblique, quadriceps strengthening, gluteus medius strengthening, and improved balance

Indications

This exercise isolates the deep local stabilizers of the knee, the vastus medialis oblique. Proper functioning of this muscle is crucial for proper patellar tracking and stabilization of the knee. It is a favorite of mine for all knee patients, as it seems that no matter what the injury is, the deep local stabilizers become inhibited. Due to the body's position for this exercise, the patient can both feel and observe proper tracking and firing of the vastus medialis oblique, making it an excellent way to retrain neuromuscularly. Since it is a unilateral weight-bearing exercise, it is also very beneficial for improving lateral hip stability (strengthening gluteus medius) and balance.

Precautions or Contraindications

Non–weight-bearing status

Resistance

Light

Instruction

Stand on the floor just in front of the foot bar, facing the carriage. Place one foot on the edge of the carriage, hooking the heel over the edge but keeping the toes pressing down against the carriage. The knee should be bent at a 90 degree angle and the kneecap aligned directly between the second and third toes. The arms are relaxed at the sides or on the hips (see photo a). Slowly push the carriage forward, bringing the leg into full knee extension (see photo b). Without moving the leg, isometrically contract the vastus medialis oblique (lower, medial part of the quadriceps) by drawing the kneecap upward. Then, slowly bend the knee and with control, return the carriage to the starting position.

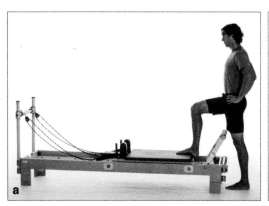
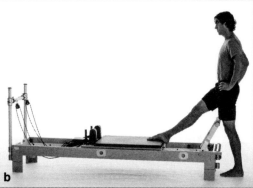
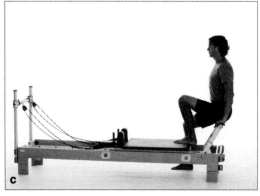
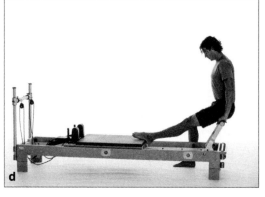

Variations

The exercise can be done half seated on the foot bar for patients of non–weight-bearing status or those having difficulty with balance (see photos c and d).

Progression

Perform the exercise standing on a balance cushion or half foam roll.

Technique Tips

1. Keep the hips even and the standing leg completely still throughout the exercise. Don't let the pelvis shift forward or back when the carriage moves.
2. Draw the core muscles in and stand up tall.
3. If having difficulty connecting with the vastus medialis oblique, touch the muscle on the inside part of the thigh just above the kneecap to feel the activation.
4. To maintain proper patellar tracking, ensure that the kneecap glides between the second and third toes when pushing the carriage out and pulling it back in.

HAMSTRING CURL

Primary Muscles Involved

Hamstrings

Objectives

Hamstring strength and proper patellar tracking

Indications

This exercise provides an easy way to target the hamstring muscles. In this position, the patient can observe the alignment and tracking of the patella, which is not possible in prone hamstring curls. The seated position also makes it appropriate for patients of non–weight-bearing status, such as after a total knee replacement surgery.

Precautions or Contraindications

This exercise is contraindicated for post-op posterior approach total hip replacement patients if the box height requires more than 90 degrees of hip flexion when in the seated position.

Resistance

Medium

Instruction

Place the short box on the reformer rails. The distance from the risers will vary depending on leg length—the shorter the legs, the closer the box will be to the carriage. Facing the foot bar, sit on the box with the legs reaching out long and hook the heels over the shoulder rests. Place the hands on the sides of the box to help hold it in place (see photo *a*). Draw the core muscles in and sit up tall. Exhale to bend the knees and pull the carriage toward the box (see photo *b*) and then inhale as the legs are straightened slowly and with control back to the starting position.

Variations

Perform the exercise one leg at a time. The other leg can be held in to the chest, resting on the box, or extended straight out to get isometric quadriceps activation.

Progression

Remove the box and do the exercise in a standing position (see photos *c* and *d*). This version is very challenging for balance and lateral hip stability, and thus great functional retraining for athletes.

Technique Tips

1. Keep the abdominals drawn in and lengthen up through the spine to stand or sit very tall.
2. Press the hands into the sides of the box, both to stabilize the box and to activate the upper body muscles.
3. To maintain proper patellar tracking, pay close attention that the kneecap glides between the second and third toes on the push out and the pull in.

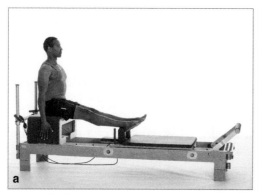
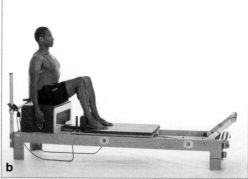
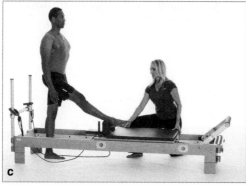
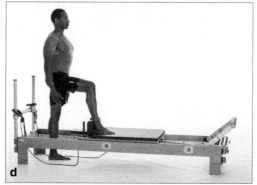

Primary Muscles Involved

Hip extensors, knee extensors, and abdominals

Objectives

Development of trunk and scapular stabilization, hip dissociation, strengthening of hip and knee extensors, and improved ability to actively contract the deep abdominals during functional activity

Indications

This is one of my favorite exercises because it is so functional and so versatile! It is a great balance exercise, and almost anyone can do it. The intention is to extend the moving leg into hip extension without compromising pelvic, trunk, and scapular stability. It is an exercise that can be easily adapted according to your objective: balance, core strength, hip extensor strength, or coordination.

Precautions or Contraindications

Lumbar disk pathology, osteoporosis, or non–weight-bearing status

Resistance

Light to medium, but heavier resistance if leg strength is the objective rather than trunk stabilization

Instruction

Stand on the floor next to the reformer, facing the foot bar. Place the hands shoulder-width apart on the foot bar with the arms straight. One foot is on the floor lined up with the shoulder rest with the knee slightly bent, and the other foot presses against the shoulder rest with the knee hovering off the carriage. Round the lower back, pull into a deep C-curve and set the core (see photo a). Inhale to push the carriage back, extending the leg that is on the carriage (see photo b). Exhale to pull the carriage back in with the abdominal muscles, bending the leg back to starting position.

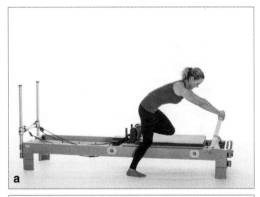

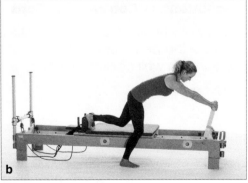

Variations

1. Patients with disk pathologies and osteoporosis should do the exercise in a neutral spine (flat back) position instead of the deep *C*-curve. This will emphasize hip extension rather than trunk flexion.
2. For elderly, immobile, or very weak clients, the supporting foot can be positioned closer to the foot bar, giving them more leverage and again favoring more toward hip extension.

Progression

Remove one hand from the foot bar and reach it forward to increase the challenge to lumbo-pelvic stability in the transverse plane.

Technique Tips

1. Avoid the tendency to round the upper back by drawing the shoulder blades down and back.
2. For the classical version, maintain lumbar flexion and posterior tilt of the pelvis throughout the exercise.
3. Imagine a runner preparing for a sprint, pushing against the starting block.

STANDING LUNGE

Primary Muscles Involved

Hamstrings and hip flexors

Objectives

Increased flexibility of the hamstrings and hip flexors

Indications

This is a great exercise to follow the scooter, as it offers a wonderful, active stretch for the hamstrings and hip flexors.

Precautions or Contraindications

Spondylolisthesis or lumbar stenosis (due to the tendency of excessive anterior tilt of the pelvis or extension of the lumbar spine in the hip flexor stretch position), as well as non–weight-bearing status

Resistance

Light

Instruction

From the scooter position (see photo *a* for the scooter exercise, p. 155), move the foot on the floor forward until it lines up with the foot bar and allow the other knee to rest on the carriage (use of a pad is recommended for sensitive knees). Exhale and slide the carriage back until a stretch is felt on the hip flexors of the leg on the carriage. Maintain a posterior tilt of the pelvis and an upright trunk. Hold the hip flexor stretch for three to five breaths (see photo *a*). Exhale to straighten the knee and lift the toes of the standing leg. Lean the chest forward toward the straight leg but keep the back straight. Hold the hamstring stretch for three to five breaths (see photo *b*).

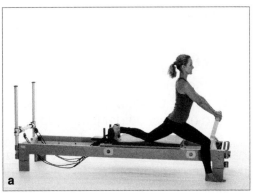

Technique Tips

1. Maintain a posterior tilt or tuck the pelvis during the hip flexor stretch.
2. Slightly anteriorly tilt the pelvis during the hamstring stretch.
3. Travel along a horizontal line with the pelvis when straightening the front leg.
4. Keep the head aligned with the spine and the back extensors engaged.

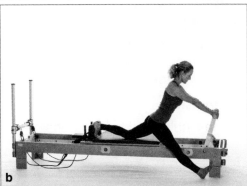

PRONE PULLING STRAPS 1

Primary Muscles Involved

Shoulder extensors and back extensors

Objectives

Shoulder and back extensor strength and improved posture

Indications

The prone position of this exercise challenges the shoulder muscles against gravity, similar to the *I*-exercise commonly prescribed in rehabilitation. The reformer straps provide additional resistance and allow for an increased challenge to the back extensors. As the entire ROM is below 90 degrees of shoulder flexion, it is safe for all shoulder pathologies and works well for adhesive capsulitis as it provides some long axis traction and thus relaxation. It is a wonderful functional exercise for swimmers and surfers as the movement is similar to paddling. The degree of extension depends on whether the objective is shoulder extension, thoracic extension, or lumbar extension.

Precautions or Contraindications

Spondylolisthesis or stenosis

Resistance

Light

Instruction

Lie prone on the long box with the sternum at the edge of the box, facing away from the foot bar, holding the ropes with the arms straight and slightly forward of the shoulder joint (approximately 20 degrees) with the palms facing in (see photo a). Inhale to lift and pull the ropes up to the sides of the body as the shoulder blades pull down the back. Lift the arms higher than the thighs if possible (see photo b). Exhale as the arms are lowered back to the starting position.

Variations

After about 5 to 10 repetitions, hold the arms up at thigh level and add triceps extensions. Bend and straighten the elbows, continuing to squeeze the shoulder blades together (see photo c).

Progression

On the inhale, add trunk extension with the shoulder extension (see photo d).

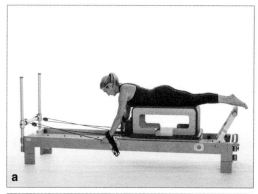
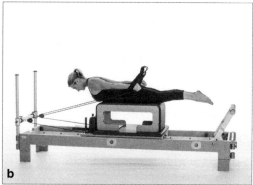
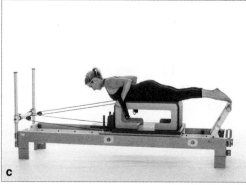
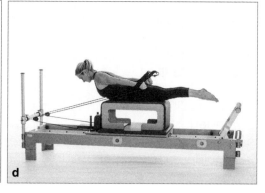

Technique Tips

1. Make sure the abdominals are engaged throughout the exercise to protect the lower back.
2. Even if not going into back extension, engage the back extensors to initiate the movement of the arms.
3. Keep the arms straight and the palms facing the reformer throughout, avoiding internal rotation of the shoulders and rounding of the chest.
4. Press the arms against the thighs at the top to activate the scapular adductors.
5. When improved posture is the goal, focus on lifting from the mid-back, arching the thoracic spine, and opening the chest (spreading wide across the collar bones and moving the shoulders down and back, as opposed to rounding the upper back and shoulders forward).
6. Keep the deep cervical flexors engaged so the cervical spine does not go into too much extension. Think of lifting the upper back, not the head and neck.

PRONE PULLING STRAPS 2

Primary Muscles Involved

Shoulder adductors and external rotators, and back extensors

Objectives

Shoulder range of motion and strength, scapular stabilization, scapulohumeral rhythm, and improved posture

Indications

As in prone pulling straps 1, the prone position of this exercise challenges the shoulder muscles against gravity, and the resistance provided by the reformer gives additional challenge to the back extensors. This one is similar to the *T* exercise commonly prescribed in rehabilitation. This is a more complex and difficult movement than pulling straps 1 because the external rotators must work to neutralize the typical pattern of internal rotation of the shoulder and rounding of the thoracic spine. This is another great exercise for swimmers and surfers, as well as anyone needing to improve posture and shoulder function.

Precautions or Contraindications

Spondylolisthesis, painful stenosis

Resistance

Light

Instruction

Lie prone on the long box facing away from the foot bar with the sternum at the edge of the box. Hold the ropes with the arms straight out to the sides in a *T* position, palms facing the floor (see photo *a*). Inhale to lift the torso and pull the shoulders down and back, bringing the arms to the sides of the body, keeping the palms facing the floor (see photo *b*). Exhale to bring the arms back to the starting position.

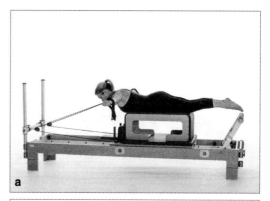

Variations

After about 5 to 10 repetitions, hold the arms in the *T* position and add scapular retraction by lifting the arms toward the ceiling against the resistance of the ropes. The carriage should not move.

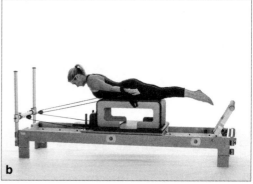

Progression

On the inhale, add trunk extension with the shoulder adduction (as in photo *d* for prone pulling straps 1 p. 158)

Technique Tips

1. Make sure the abdominals are engaged throughout the exercise to protect the lower back.
2. Even if not going into back extension, engage the back extensors to initiate the movement of the arms.
3. Ensure external rotation of the shoulders by keeping the palms facing the floor throughout the motion. Bring the little fingers (rather than the palms or the thumb) to touch the thighs.
4. Move the arms along a horizontal plane, staying parallel to the floor as the shoulders abduct and adduct.
5. When improved posture is the goal, focus on lifting from the mid-back, arching the thoracic spine, and opening the chest.
6. Keep the deep cervical flexors engaged so the cervical spine does not go into too much extension. Think of lifting the upper back, not the head and neck.

QUADRATUS LUMBORUM STRETCH

Primary Muscles Involved

Quadratus lumborum

Objectives

Stretch the quadratus lumborum

Indications

This is a wonderful, passive stretch of the very often tight quadratus lumborum. This muscle is often the source of low back pain and can be difficult to stretch effectively. The design of the reformer puts the client into a great stretch position where manual assist and mobilization can easily be added.

Precautions or Contraindications

Lumbar disk pathologies or osteoporosis (part 2 only)

Resistance

Heavy (all springs)

Instruction

Move the spring bar forward and grab the foot strap underneath, then return the spring bar to the appropriate position. The spring bar should be positioned farthest away from the foot bar for a taller person and closest to the foot bar for a shorter person. Attach all springs and place the box on the reformer, perpendicular to it. Sit sideways on the box, bend the leg farthest from the foot bar and place that hip on the back edge of the box. Hook the foot of the top leg underneath the foot strap and make sure it is secure (see photo a). Part 1: Side bend away from the foot bar and place either the hand or the elbow on the headrest (depending on flexibility and torso length). Reach the upper arm overhead until a stretch is felt and hold for three to five breaths (see photo b). Part 2: If appropriate, rotate the trunk toward the floor and place one hand on each rail. Lower the trunk until a stretch is felt and hold for three to five breaths (see photo c).

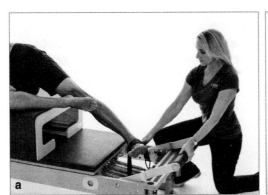
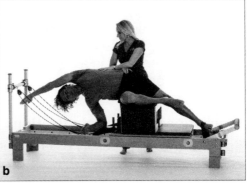

Variations

Instructor can apply manual myofascial release or soft tissue mobilization as the patient stretches in this position.

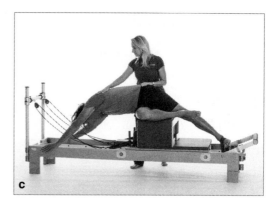

Progression

More flexible or taller people can place the hand on the floor.

Technique Tips

1. Make sure the hips are stacked so that it is a pure side bend without any twisting of the spine (for part 1).
2. Make sure the leg of the foot that is hooked under the foot strap is completely straight and that there is tension on the strap in order to get the full benefit of the stretch. Move the spring bar to a different position if necessary to accommodate this.
3. In both positions, the body should be completely relaxed and drape over the box, letting gravity and the stabilization of the foot strap create a passive stretch.

JUMPING SERIES

Primary Muscles Involved

Quadriceps and gastrocnemius

Objectives

Knee extensor strength, hip extensor strength, plantar flexor strength, lumbopelvic stabilization, and neuromuscular reeducation for running and jumping

Indications

The jump board attachment provides a great functional retraining exercise for athletes. Jumping on the reformer allows for earlier progressive load bearing using zero-gravity spring resistance. This allows for exact functional patterns and muscle memory to be retrained so that when the patient is ready to return to his sport, the motion has already been learned and the correct muscles strengthened. It is also a great way to help someone with poor landing mechanics learn proper deceleration techniques, and it is a great challenge for the core!

Precautions or Contraindications

Spinal and lower extremity osteoarthritis in which impact is not recommended; acute lower extremity injuries such as patellar tendinitis, iliotibial band syndrome, Achilles tendinitis, posterior tibialis tendinitis, plantar fasciitis, or ankle sprain

Resistance

Light to medium

Instruction

Insert and secure the jump board according to equipment guidelines. Lie supine in a neutral spine position on the reformer, legs parallel and feet on the jump board, hip-width apart, and heels pressing down (see photo *a*). Exhale to straighten the knees, plantar flex the feet, and jump off the board (see photo *b*). Inhale to return to the starting position, allowing the knees to bend and the heels to slowly descend back to the board. Repeat 10 to 20 times, keeping the core engaged so the carriage does not move.

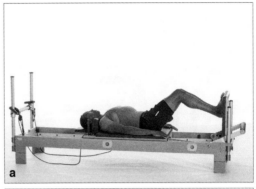

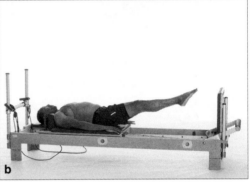

Variations

1. *V position:* This variation has the same setup and movement as the main exercise, but with the legs externally rotated and the feet on the board in a *V* position, heels pressing down (see photo *c*). Squeeze the legs together when in the air to work the adductors and land with the knees aligned over the second and third toes. Repeat 10 to 20 times.

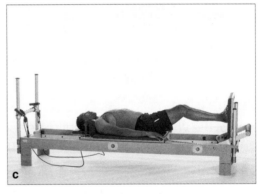

2. *Unilateral:* In this variation, start with one foot on the board as in the bilateral version, but with the other leg held in the tabletop position (see photo *d*). Jump and land on the same leg 10 times. Then switch legs.

3. *Leg changes (skipping):* This variation is the same as the unilateral variation, but as the jumping leg straightens, the opposite leg also straightens. Switch legs in the air and land on the opposite leg, allowing the knee to bend with the impact as the other leg is held in the tabletop position (see photo *e*).

4. *Extended knees (hopping):* In this variation, keep the knees extended during both the jump and the landing (see photos *f* and *g*). This version works the lower leg muscles rather than the quadriceps, making it very

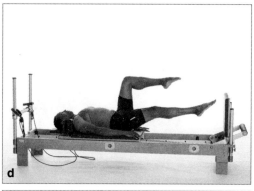
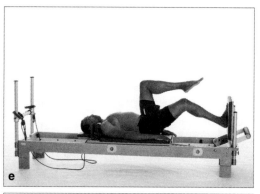
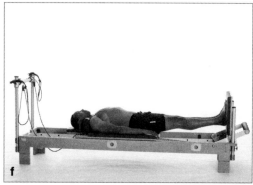
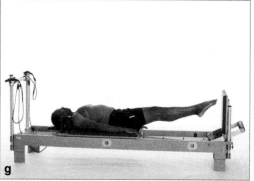

valuable for recovery and prevention of injuries such as chronic ankle sprain or Achilles tendinosis. It is also excellent for helping older people in fall prevention as it trains the neuromuscular system to be able to generate force or torque rapidly, without a lot of load to stress the joints.

Progression

Any of the variations or the entire sequence can be performed while catching and throwing a ball or lifting small hand weights.

Technique Tips

1. If the core muscles are not engaged, all the force comes from the legs, and this causes the carriage to move. Do not allow this to happen. If it is impossible to prevent, lighten the springs until the correct muscle patterning is learned to achieve the motion while the carriage remains still.
2. Strive to maintain heel contact following the landing without a double bounce.
3. Articulate through the foot on push-off and landing, just as one would do for running or jumping.
4. The push-off should be dynamic, but the landing very soft and controlled.
5. In the unilateral versions, keep the pelvis stable and level and the tabletop leg completely still.

7

Cadillac Exercises

The Cadillac, though large and quite expensive, is a very useful apparatus to have in a rehab setting. The height and width make it very user friendly and safe for elderly or frail clients, and for those with postsurgical range-of-motion restrictions. It is also very stable, which is great for people who are uncomfortable with the moving platform of the reformer. It can also be used as a plinth for joint and soft-tissue mobilization, proprioceptive neuromuscular facilitation, or manual stretching. Due to its design, it challenges the body in multiple planes of motion. As with the reformer and wunda chair, exercises can be done in prone, supine, side-lying, sitting, kneeling, and standing positions on the apparatus. There are also some wonderful functional exercises that are done standing on the floor next to the Cadillac, using its springs or bars for resistance or support. Regarding safety, extra caution must be used when using the push-through bar (PTB) on the Cadillac. If it is suddenly released when top-loaded, it pops up very quickly and can strike the instructor or client. Use of the safety strap when doing exercises that require a bottom-loaded PTB is necessary.

Each Cadillac exercise is described with detailed instruction, primary muscles involved, objectives, indications, precautions or contraindications, variations and progressions as appropriate, and technique tips for correct execution. In addition, suggested setup and spring resistance is given. The exercise instructions are written in a voice such that a professional can instruct his or her patient or client, and such that the directions can be followed by the practitioner him or herself. I recommend that anyone who does not have experience with Pilates works with a certified instructor to practice the exercises—both in the role of the client and of the teacher—before applying them in a rehabilitation practice. This is essential in being able to provide a safe and effective exercise program.

PELVIC CURL WITH ROLL-UP BAR

*A variation of an original exercise taught by Rael Isacowitz in the BASI Master II Program (Isacowitz 2018).

Primary Muscles Involved

Abdominals, hamstrings, and gluteus maximus

Objectives

Mobilization of the spine and pelvic region, spinal articulation, hamstring control, pelvic lumbar stabilization, recruitment and cocontraction of the core muscles, and mild spinal traction

Indications

This exercise is simply a pelvic curl on the mat (p. 57) with the roll-up bar (RUB) placed under the knees. This provides a bit of spinal traction and aids in releasing the hip flexors. The addition of resistance helps people who have difficulty articulating through a pelvic curl, such as those with general stiffness or arthritis of the spine, weak or inhibited core, or tightness of back extensors or hip flexors. It is a great way to begin a Pilates session as it promotes relaxation and the mind–body connection, and it gets the spine moving and primed for more challenging exercises.

Precautions or Contraindications

Acute lumbar disk pathology or osteoporosis (due to the deep spinal flexion)

Resistance

Medium (two blue or red springs on RUB attached at approximately three-quarters height)

Instructions

Lie supine on the Cadillac with bent knees, legs parallel approximately hip-distance apart, arms relaxed at the sides with palms down, and pelvis in a neutral position. Hook the RUB under the knees with moderate tension on the springs (see photo a). Inhale to prepare and exhale to set the core and

begin to curl the pelvis and spine off the mat, one vertebra at a time (see photo b). Inhale to hold at the top of the ROM, where the pelvis should be at maximum posterior tilt and a stretch should be felt in the hip flexors. Exhale as the spine is lowered, starting in the thoracic spine and rolling down one vertebra at a time until the tailbone touches the mat.

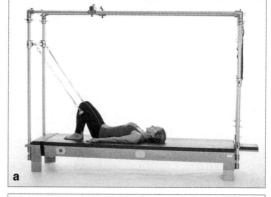

a

Variations

1. For patients with disk pathologies, omit the deep lumbar flexion and simply maintain the spine and pelvis in a neutral position as it is lifted.

2. Place a ball between the knees to promote more adductor engagement.

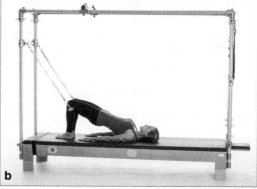

b

Progression

1. Reach the arms overhead as the pelvis lifts to elicit more upper spine control (see photos *c* and *d*).
2. Bottom lift on reformer (p. 94) and bottom lift with extension on reformer (p. 95).

Technique Tips

1. Keep the neck and shoulders relaxed.
2. Maximize lumbar flexion as the spine lifts off the mat by pulling the pubic bone towards the chin (posteriorly tilting the pelvis).
3. Think of pulling the heels toward the tailbone to keep the hamstrings engaged and the pelvis posteriorly tilted.
4. Visualize the lowering of the spine like a Slinky spring toy going down steps, deliberately placing one vertebra at a time. This will help to achieve maximum articulation and spinal mobility.

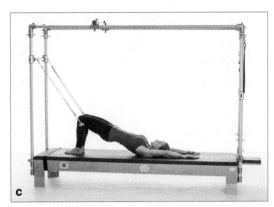

c

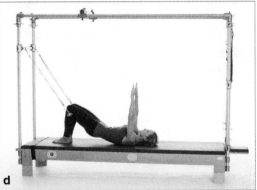

d

BREATHING WITH PUSH-THROUGH BAR

Primary Muscles Involved

Abdominals and back extensors

Objectives

Abdominal strength, spinal articulation and mobility, shoulder mobility, and improved coordination, balance, and breathing

Indications

As discussed in chapters 2 and 3, the basic breath pattern used in BASI Pilates is to exhale with spinal flexion and inhale with spinal extension. This is an excellent exercise to teach this concept of coordination of breath and movement. The body moves fluidly through shoulder flexion and extension, lumbar flexion, lumbar and thoracic extension, and hip flexion and extension. The springs provide assistance for those who have restricted mobility or core strength and usually cannot reach these positions.

Precautions or Contraindications

Acute disk pathology, acute sacroiliac joint dysfunction or pain, or acute shoulder impingement

Resistance

Medium (two blue or one red spring) or less to increase the challenge

Instructions

Lie supine on the Cadillac in a neutral pelvis position with the feet resting on the trapeze strap and the hands holding the PTB with the arms shoulder-width apart. The legs should be straight with the feet externally rotated and the shoulders at 90 degrees of flexion (see photo *a*). Inhale and pull the PTB back overhead (see photo *b*). Exhale and return the bar to the starting position. Inhale to draw the abdominals in and curl the pelvis and spine up into a bridge position (see photo *c*). Exhale and lower the spine and pelvis back to the mat, one vertebra at a time. Inhale to draw the abdominals in and roll up into a teaser position (see photo *d*). Exhale and roll back down to the starting position.

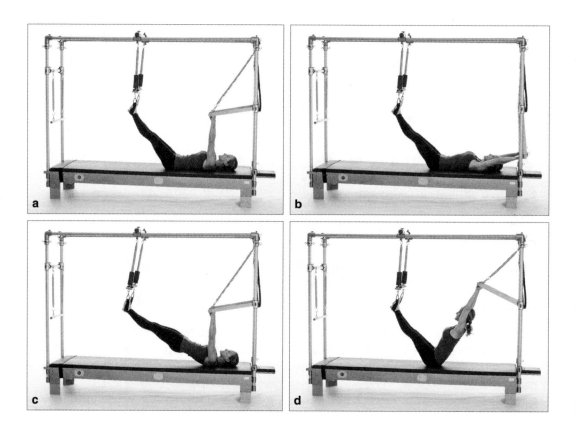

Variations

When patients with disk pathologies lift into the bridge position, they should do so in a neutral spine position (flat back) and hinge up rather than rolling up. Doing the exercise this way will emphasize hip extension rather than deep abdominal activation.

Progression

Perform the exercise with the feet supported by a large physio ball rather than the trapeze strap. This version is more difficult because it challenges lumbo-pelvic stability in multiple planes.

Technique Tips

1. Coordinate the movement with the breath and keep both fluid.
2. Keep the spine in a neutral position and avoid flaring the ribs when reaching the bar overhead.
3. In the teaser position (photo *d* in breathing with push-through bar, p. 168), reach the chest toward the feet and strive to make the spine as long as possible, allowing the bar to provide slight traction.

HIP WORK: DOUBLE LEG SUPINE

This series is another great way to teach the concept of hip dissociation, as well as to increase hip joint mobility and correct any muscular imbalances in the hip region. Imbalances in hip musculature are often the cause of lumbar, pelvic, hip, and even knee pathologies. This series addresses these imbalances, as the primary muscles worked are the hip extensors and adductors rather than the often too-tight hip flexors. It is similar to the hip work on the reformer series (p. 108), but because of the angle of resistance there is more load on the hip extensors. Unlike the reformer, on the Cadillac each leg uses a separate spring, which makes them work completely independent of one another, thus increasing the challenge of pelvic stability and enhancing the ability to detect any imbalances between sides. I like using the Cadillac for patients with instability, balance, or coordination issues (for example neurological pathologies such as stroke, multiple sclerosis, or fibromyalgia) because it promotes a feeling of stability. Because the Cadillac is higher than the reformer, it is easier and safer to get on and off. This is especially valuable for early post-op total hip replacement (THR) patients as the contraindication of no more than 90 degrees of hip flexion precaution is inherently respected. This series is also great for patients with sacroiliac joint dysfunction. As on the reformer, the range can be increased or decreased according to the patient's ability or limitations.

FROG

Primary Muscles Involved

Hip adductors

Objectives

Lumbo-pelvic stability, hip dissociation, hip mobility, adductor strength and control, and knee extensor control

Indications

This is a great exercise for stiff or arthritic hips and knees, sacroiliac joint pathologies, and anyone needing to develop pelvic-lumbar stabilization.

Precautions or Contraindications

Use caution with post-op total hip joint replacement patients, as the tendency is to go into >90 hip flexion when the legs pull in to the frog position.

Resistance

Leg springs are attached to the crossbar approximately three fourths of the way up the poles. Use the light (yellow) leg springs to orient the work toward lumbo-pelvic stabilization. Resistance can be increased (purple leg springs) if the objective is strengthening the hip extensors or adductors.

Instruction

Lie supine in a neutral pelvis position on the Cadillac with the feet in the straps, knees bent into the frog position with the feet dorsi flexed. The arms are by the sides with the shoulders relaxed (see photo *a*). Exhale and squeeze the heels together, pushing the legs straight along a horizontal line (see photo *b*). Inhale and return to the starting position.

Variation

The straps can be placed above the knees to decrease the lever arm for severe instability or neurological pathologies.

Progression

Frog can be done with one leg in the strap (called hip work: single leg supine), while the other is straight out on the mat (see photo *c*).

Technique Tips

1. Initiate the movement with the hamstrings and adductors.
2. Focus on squeezing the legs together as the knees straighten, as if holding a balloon between the legs.
3. Glue the heels together throughout the exercise, especially when straightening out to full knee extension.
4. Move the feet along a consistent horizontal plane.

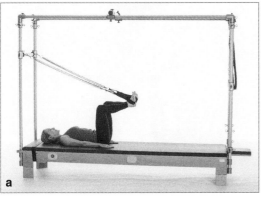

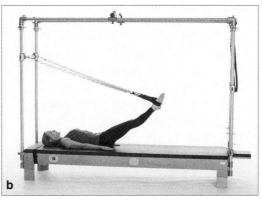

5. Keep the pelvis stable through-out the exercise.

6. Avoid bringing the knees too close to the chest, as this can cause the tailbone to lift and makes the exercise contraindi-cated for post-op THR.

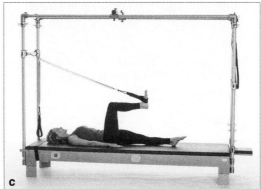

HIP CIRCLES

Primary Muscles Involved

Hip adductors and hip extensors

Objectives

Lumbo-pelvic stabilization; hip mobility; hip adductor, abductor, and extensor strength and control; hip dissociation; and adductor and hamstring muscle elongation

Indications

This is a fabulous exercise for adductor control and strength as they are forced to work isometrically, concentrically, and eccentrically. This is one of my favorite exercises for developing hip dissociation and increasing hip joint ROM.

Precautions or Contraindications

None

Resistance

Leg springs are attached to the crossbar approximately three fourths of the way up the poles. Use the light (yellow) leg springs to orient the work toward lumbo-pelvic stabilization. Resistance can be increased (purple leg springs) if the objective is strengthening the hip extensors or adductors.

Instruction

Lie supine on the Cadillac in a neutral pelvis position with the feet in the straps, legs straight, hips at 90 degrees of flexion (if possible without tilting the pelvis). Externally rotate the hips and plantar flex the feet. The arms are by the sides with the shoulders relaxed (see photo *a*). Exhale and draw the legs straight down the midline, keeping them pressed together (see photo *b*) and then inhale and open the legs (see photo *c*), circling them around and back up to the starting position. Repeat 5 to 10 times and then reverse direction.

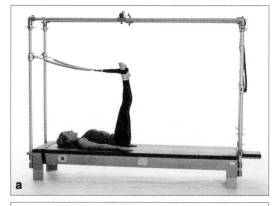

Variation

The straps can be placed above the knees to decrease the lever arm for severe instability or neurological pathologies.

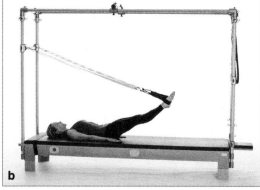

Progression

The progression for this exercise is the same as for frog (p. 170), with one leg in the strap (called hip work: single leg supine) and the other straight out on the mat.

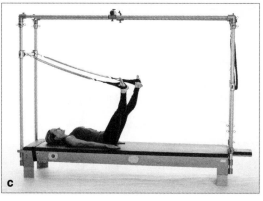

Technique Tips

1. Imagine drawing a circular shape on the ceiling, maintaining tension in the springs throughout the movement.
2. Squeeze the legs together as they draw a line up or down the center.
3. Engage the hamstrings with the adductors by squeezing in as well as pushing down against an imaginary balloon as the legs are lowered down the center.
4. Maximize the contraction of the adductors when opening and closing the legs.
5. Focus on pelvic stability as well as hip dissociation.

WALKING

Primary Muscles Involved

Hip extensors

Objectives

Lumbo-pelvic stability, hip joint mobility, hip extensor strength, and hip dissociation

Indications

This exercise reinforces pelvic stability with hip mobility in the sagittal plane. It is effective in showing patients where in their range of motion they start to lose their neutral spine position and which muscles they can use to control this. The starting position elicits initiation of leg movement from the hamstrings, while at the same time giving these muscles an active stretch. It is adaptable for all, as the range can be increased or decreased according to the patient's abilities or limitations.

Resistance

Leg springs are attached to the crossbar approximately three fourths of the way up the poles. Use the light (yellow) leg springs to orient the work toward lumbo-pelvic stabilization. Resistance can be increased (purple leg springs) if the objective is strengthening the hip extensors or adductors.

Precautions or Contraindications

None

Instruction

Lie supine on the Cadillac in a neutral pelvis position with the feet in the straps, legs squeezing straight and parallel, hips at 90 degrees of flexion (if possible without tilting the pelvis). The arms are by the sides with the shoulders relaxed (see photo a). Exhale and alternate the legs with a small scissor-like motion while extending the hips and pressing the legs down toward the mat for five counts (see photo b). Inhale and raise the legs back up to the starting position while resisting the springs with the same scissor-like motion for five counts.

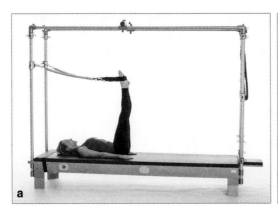
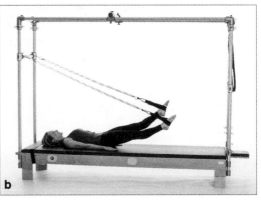

Variation

The straps can be placed above the knees to decrease the lever arm for severe instability or neurological pathologies.

Progression

As for frog and circles (p. 170 and p. 180) perform with one leg in the strap while the other is straight out on the mat (called hip work: single leg supine). The leg in the strap

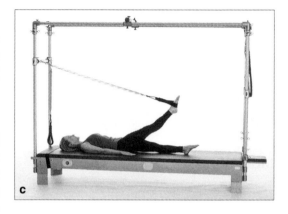

pulls down into hip extension, maximizing work for the hamstrings while the pelvis and opposite leg remain stable (see photo c).

Technique Tips

1. Keep the leg movements small and controlled, as if swimming with flutter kicks.
2. Keep tension in the springs throughout the exercise.
3. Focus on lumbo-pelvic stability.

SUPINE HIP FLEXOR STRETCH WITH MANUAL ASSIST

Primary Muscles Involved

Hip flexors

Objective

Release and increase the flexibility of the hip flexors

Indications

This is a safe, comfortable way to stretch for anyone who has tight hip flexors. The downward pressure provided by the crossbar prevents the lumbar spine from going into hyperextension, which is what normally occurs with this stretch. A common remedy for this is to hold the knee of the non-stretching leg to the chest, but this forces other muscles to engage and thus prevents the release of tension and the ability to get the maximum benefit out of the stretch. The design of the Cadillac, along with some manual assistance, allows one to enjoy a completely passive stretch of the hip flexors.

Precautions or Contraindications

Contraindications include early stages post-op posterior approach THR (due to nonstretching leg position of >90 degrees hip flexion). Use caution with spondylolisthesis.

Resistance

None

Instructions

Lie supine at the RUB end of the Cadillac, with the tailbone at the edge of the mat. Bend one knee in toward the chest and let the other leg hang off the edge, with the arms relaxed at the sides (see photo *a*). The instructor lowers the crossbar to the appropriate height for patient comfort and places the bar on the plantar surface of the patient's foot. The instructor then half kneels on the floor and presses the patient's stretching leg gently and slowly into hip extension and knee flexion until the patient reports that a good stretch is felt (see photo *b*). Hold for a few breaths, and then lift the patient's stretching leg up and place the foot under the bar next to the opposite foot. Repeat the stretch on the opposite side.

Technique Tips

1. To get in and out of the position, simply raise the crossbar and have the patient use the poles for assistance moving from sitting to supine.
2. Make sure that the crossbar provides enough downward pressure to keep the patient's spine pressing into the mat.
3. Dorsi flex the foot on the bar, with the plantar surface facing the ceiling.
4. If the patient doesn't feel the stretch, have him slide farther off the edge of the Cadillac so the hip is in more of an extended position.

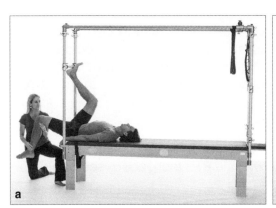 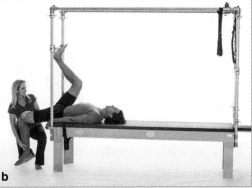

SUPINE PROTRACTION AND RETRACTION ON FOAM ROLL

Primary Muscles Involved

Serratus anterior, rhomboids, and middle trapezius

Objectives

Scapular protraction and retraction strength and scapular mobility

Indications

A weak serratus anterior (SA) is a very common finding in people with shoulder pathologies. This exercise is a great way to isolate and strengthen the SA, which is so important in proper shoulder function, especially in athletes. The primary role of the SA is to stabilize the scapula during elevation and to pull the scapula forward and around on the thoracic cage, as needed in swimming, pushing, punching, or throwing. As discussed in chapter 3, research has shown that the SA and lower trapezius (LT) are the most commonly weak or inhibited muscles of the scapulothoracic joint that may lead to abnormal movement. Thus, it is crucial in our shoulder patients to strengthen this muscle. This exercise provides an easy way to isolate the SA so patients can learn what it feels like to activate it and can then properly do so in more challenging exercises and sporting activities.

Precautions or Contraindications

None

Resistance

Heavy (two bottom loaded red springs on the PTB)

Instructions

Lie supine on a half foam roll holding the bottom-loaded PTB (safety strap on!), with the hands directly over the shoulders. Bend the knees and place the feet flat on the mat, with the spine in a neutral position and the foam roll in between the shoulder blades (see photo a). Exhale to protract the scapulae by pressing the bar up against resistance with straight arms (see photo b). Inhale and lower the bar, pulling the scapulae into retraction with the arms remaining straight.

Variations

If the objective is to strengthen scapular retraction (rhomboids and middle trapezius), perform the same exercise but with the PTB top loaded (see photo c).

Progression

1. To challenge core stability, perform the exercise on a full foam roll.
2. Perform the exercise unilaterally (see photo d).

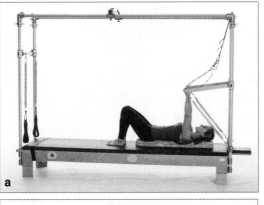
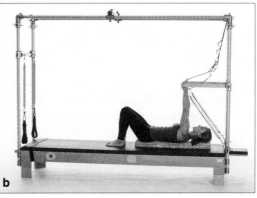
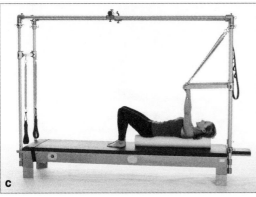
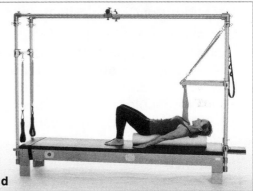

Technique Tips

1. Keep the elbows completely straight throughout the exercises.
2. Keep the abdominals engaged and the body stable.
3. As the bar is pulled down, squeeze the shoulder blades around the foam roll.
4. Keep the chin slightly tucked to engage the deep neck flexors.
5. Keep the LT engaged and not let the shoulders elevate toward the ears.

SINGLE-LEG SIDE SERIES

This series offers the same benefits as the hip work: double leg supine series (p. 169). Because this series takes place in the side-lying position, the hip abductors and obliques are also recruited.

CHANGES

Primary Muscles Involved

Hip adductors

Objectives

Adductor strength and control and lumbo-pelvic stabilization

Indications

This is a fabulous exercise for adductor control and strength as these muscles are forced to work isometrically, concentrically, and eccentrically. It is effective in showing patients where in their range of motion they start to lose their neutral spine position and which muscles they can use to control this. It is adaptable for all, as the range of motion can be increased or decreased according to the patient's ability or limitations.

Precautions or Contraindications

Contraindications include greater trochanteric bursitis, and early post-op posterior approach THR (due to hip adduction past midline). For shoulder impingement syndrome, the arm position can be modified.

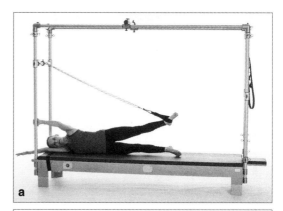

Resistance

Light to medium (yellow leg spring from three quarters up pole or from the top of the frame for more resistance)

Instructions

Lie sideways on the Cadillac with the legs straight and externally rotated. The top leg reaches out in a diagonal line (approximately 45 degrees) with the foot in the strap (see photo a). The bottom arm is straight overhead with the head resting on the arm as the top arm holds the side pole or simply rests on the Cadillac in front of the body. Exhale and lower the top leg in front of the bottom leg (see photo b), then inhale and lift the top leg. Exhale to lower the top leg and touch it down behind the bottom leg (see photo c), then inhale to lift the top leg back to the starting positon.

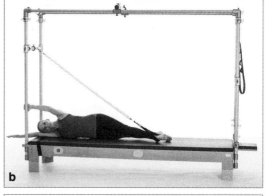

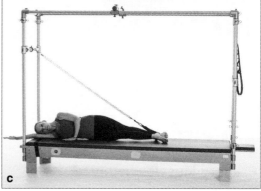

Variations

1. The strap can be placed above the knees to decrease the lever arm for severe instability or neurological pathologies.
2. For shoulder or neck pathologies, a pillow can be used to support the head and the arms can be placed in a comfortable position.

Technique Tips

1. Draw in the abdominals with particular focus on the obliques to create and maintain a small space under the waist throughout the exercise.
2. Minimize movement at the pelvis, keeping the top hip stacked directly over the bottom hip.
3. Imagine both legs reaching out from the hip sockets.

SCISSORS

Primary Muscles Involved

Hip extensors and hip flexors

Objectives

Hip extensor strength and control, hip flexor stretch, and lumbo-pelvic stabilization

Indications

This exercise reinforces pelvic stability with hip mobility in the sagittal plane, similar to walking (p. 173) but because it is done in the side-lying position the adductors, abductors and obliques are more involved. An additional benefit of this position is that the legs can go into hip extension past neutral, thereby creating a hip flexor stretch. It is effective in showing patients where in their range of motion they start to lose their neutral spine position and which muscles they can use to control this. It is adaptable for all, as the range can be increased or decreased according to the patient's ability or limitations.

Precautions or Contraindications

Contraindications include greater trochanteric bursitis. For shoulder impingement syndrome, the arm position can be modified.

Resistance

Light to medium (yellow leg spring three quarters of the way up the pole or from the top of the frame for more resistance)

Instructions

Lie sideways on the Cadillac with the legs straight, externally rotated, and pressing together. The top foot is in the strap (see photo *a*). The bottom arm is straight overhead with the head resting on the arm and the top arm holds the side pole or simply rests on the Cadillac in front of the body (see photo *a*). Exhale and bring the top leg forward while reaching the bottom leg back, keeping both legs straight for two pulses (two small movements) (see photo *b*). Inhale and switch legs for two pulses.

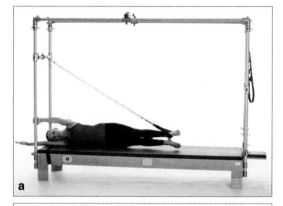

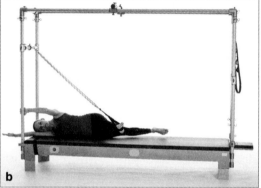

Variations

The variations for this series are the same as for single-leg side series—changes (p. 177).

Technique Tips

1. The tips for single-leg side series—changes (p. 177) also apply here.
2. Move the top and bottom legs through equal ranges of motion to maintain pelvic and hip stability.
3. Strive to feel a hip flexor stretch when the leg reaches back.

CIRCLES (FORWARD AND BACK)

Primary Muscles Involved

Hip adductors, extensors, and flexors

Objectives

Lumbo-pelvic stabilization; hip mobility; hip adductor, abductor, flexor, and extensor strength and control; hip dissociation; and hip muscle elongation

Indications

The indications for this exercise are the same as for hip circles from the hip work: double leg supine series (p. 171), but with the additional benefit of reaching the leg past midline into hip extension and therefore getting a hip flexor stretch.

Precautions or Contraindications

Contraindications include greater trochanteric bursitis. For shoulder impingement syndrome, the arm position can be modified.

Resistance

Light to medium (yellow leg spring three quarters of the way up the pole or from the top of the frame for more resistance)

Instructions

Lie sideways on the Cadillac with the legs straight, externally rotated, and pressing together. Place the top foot in the strap. The bottom arm is straight overhead with the head resting on the arm and the top arm holds the side pole or simply rests on the Cadillac in front of the body (see photo a). Inhale and reach the top leg forward (see photo b). Exhale and circle the leg up, around, and back, then return to the starting position (see photo c and d). Repeat 5 to 10 times and then switch direction.

Variations

The variations for this series are the same as for the single-leg side series—changes (p. 177).

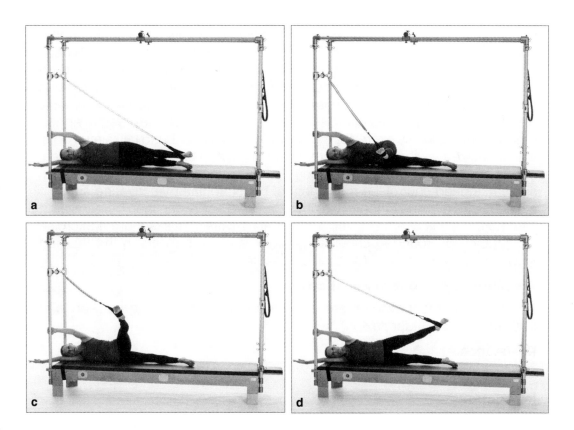

Technique Tips

1. The tips for single-leg side series—changes (p. 177) also apply here.
2. Maintain tension in the spring throughout the entire circle.
3. Maximize external rotation of the hip throughout.
4. Strive to feel a hip flexor stretch when the leg reaches back.

SEATED PROTRACTION AND RETRACTION (MODIFICATION OF SHOULDER ADDUCTION SITTING FORWARD)

Primary Muscles Involved

Latissimus dorsi and lower and middle trapezius

Objectives

Scapular adduction and depression strength and control, scapular mobility, and stability

Indications

This exercise provides neuromuscular retraining and increases mobility for people who have difficulty moving the scapula or isolating the scapular stabilizing muscles. It is very common, especially in people suffering from neck or shoulder pathologies, that the upper trapezius is over-recruited, causing elevated shoulders and neck tension. The scapulae tend to get stuck in one position and become hypermobile or stiff. The LT is one of the most commonly weak or inhibited muscles of the scapulothoracic joint that may lead to abnormal movement. In this exercise, the ability to recruit the LT and latissimus dorsi is emphasized, as the scapulae are drawn down and back against resistance. In this comfortable position with very little resistance, the client learns that she can indeed control the movement of her scapulae by activating specific muscles and relaxing others. This newly learned ability can then be translated into more difficult exercises and functional activities. This is a great exercise for people with rounded shoulder posture, and for patients in the thawing stages of frozen shoulder (adhesive capsulitis).

Precautions or Contraindications

Acute impingement syndrome or adhesive capsulitis (starting position is at >90 degrees shoulder flexion)

Resistance

Medium (two blue arm springs on PTB)

Instructions

Sit upright in a straddle position on the Cadillac with one hand pressing into each side of the PTB with the arms straight and with soft elbows (not hyperex-

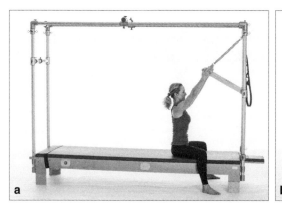 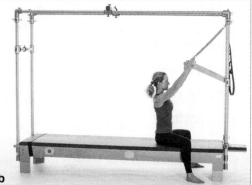

tended) (see photo *a*). Exhale to retract and depress the scapulae by drawing the PTB down and back without bending the elbows (see photo *b*). Inhale and resist as the bar pulls the arms back to the starting position.

Variations

Classically, this exercise is performed by bending the elbows to draw the bar down. Doing so, however, moves the focus from the LT to the biceps.

Technique Tips

1. Sit up tall, with the pelvis in as close to a neutral position as possible.
2. When drawing the bar down, think of putting the shoulder blades in the back pants pockets.
3. Actively resist the bar returning to the starting position to create some activation of the SA.
4. Avoid elevation of the shoulders as the bar returns to the starting position.

PUSH-THROUGH SITTING STRETCHES

Primary Muscles Involved

Hamstrings and spinal extensors

Objectives

Spinal mobility and traction, hamstring stretch, lower back stretch, and latissimus dorsi stretch

Indications

This exercise is a wonderful way to stretch and mobilize patients with a tight back. The design of the Cadillac puts the patient into a great stretch position where manual assist, mobilization, and traction can easily be added by the instructor.

Precautions or Contraindications

Lumbar disk pathologies and osteoporosis or early stages post-op posterior approach THR (due to >90 degrees hip flexion position)

Resistance

Medium (one or two red arm springs on PTB)

Instructions

The patient sits on the Cadillac facing the PTB, feet pressing against the side poles, hands on the PTB shoulder-width apart. The instructor kneels on the Cadillac behind the patient.

Part 1

On an inhale, the patient pulls the bar in by engaging the abdominals and leaning back slightly, then pushes the bar forward into a forward flexion stretch position. Hold this stretch for 3-5 breath cycles. Instructor can apply manual stretching and/or joint and soft tissue mobilization (see photo *a*).

Part 2

On an inhale the patient pulls PTB back toward him and then exhales to press it up to the ceiling. The instructor stands and places one knee against the patient's back at the appropriate level and applies pressure up and forward. At the same time, the instructor uses both hands to press up against the PTB, assisting the bar in providing spinal traction. Hold stretch for 3-5 breath cycles (see photo *b*).

Part 3

The patient pulls the PTB back to starting position as he inhales and then rotates the upper body while reaching one hand to the opposite side pole as he exhales. The instructor half kneels and presses one knee against the patient's side-reaching shoulder, facilitating spinal rotation with gentle pressure. The instructor pushes the PTB up to apply traction with one hand, while

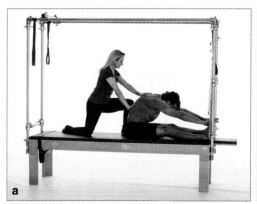
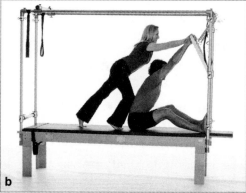

the other hand and forearm supports the patient's arm that is on the PTB, gently encouraging more rotation. Hold the stretch for three to five breath cycles (see photo *c*) and then repeat on the other side.

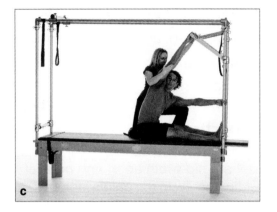
c

Variations

These stretches can be done with bent knees, sitting on a pad or small box, or even in a straddle position for those with tight hamstrings.

Technique Tips

1. In all phases, think of lengthening the spine rather than compressing.
2. Keep the abdominals engaged to protect the lower back, especially in part 1.
3. In part 2, think of reaching the chest forward and lengthening through the spine to grow as tall as possible.
4. In part 3, the more surface area contact you have with the patient, the more stable and secure he will feel. Rather than just holding the patient's arm distally, get in close and use the entire forearm.

ASSISTED SQUATS

Primary Muscles Involved

Quadriceps, glutes, and biceps

Objectives

Lower extremity strength and stability and decreased load on hip and knee joints during functional movement

Indications

The heavy springs from above provide resistance to unload the hip and knee joints (decrease joint compression and the amount of weight bearing), allowing the patient to perform the functional movement of a squat with less joint compression. This makes it a wonderful exercise for arthritic hips and knees. Because it is done in an upright position as opposed to the forward flexed position of a typical squat, neutral alignment is encouraged and load on the lower back is decreased. It is also a great exercise for clients with generalized weakness, for example from a stroke or advanced age, because the springs provide some stability and allow accomplishment of the movement and neuromuscular patterning. If the objective is to challenge lower extremity strength and balance for an athlete, this exercise can be progressed by decreasing the resistance or moving to a single-leg version.

Precautions or Contraindications

Non–weight-bearing status or severe hip or knee osteoarthritis

Resistance

Very heavy (two red arm springs) when the objective is to unload the joints; light to medium when the objective is to challenge strength, stability and balance

Instructions

Stand on the floor facing the upright poles on the RUB side of the Cadillac. The feet are hip-width apart and parallel. Hold the RUB in both hands, shoulder-width apart with the palms facing up and elbows bent slightly so there is some tension in the springs (see photo a). Exhale and bend the knees to go into a squat position (with the knees over the ankles and the back straight) as the elbows bend to 90 degrees, performing a biceps curl (see photo b). Inhale to straighten the knees and return to the starting position.

Variations

The biceps curl (bending the arms from straight to 90 degrees flexion) can be omitted if necessary due to upper extremity pathology or lack of coordination.

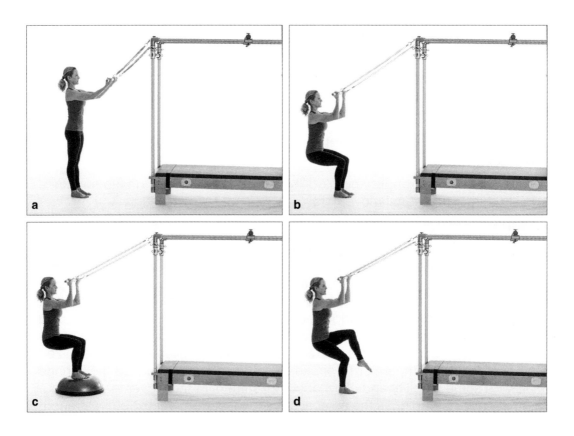

Progression

1. Instead of the RUB, attach the handles to the springs. This decreases stability and thus increases the challenge.
2. To further increase the challenge, attach the springs to the crossbar instead of the top rails. The lower the crossbar, the less resistance provided by the springs, which will increase the load on the knee and hip joints.
3. Perform the exercise on a BOSU ball or balance pad (see photo *c*).
4. To further challenge balance and strength, perform a single leg squat in any of the previous positions (see photo *d*).

Technique Tips

1. Maintain proper tracking of the knees throughout the exercise (the kneecaps should be aligned directly over the second and third toes).
2. Reach the hips back as if attempting to sit in a chair, ensuring that the knees are directly over the ankles (not the toes) when squatting.
3. Keep the trunk upright as if sliding up and down against a wall.

RESISTED LUNGES

Primary Muscles Involved

Quadriceps and glutes

Objectives

Lower extremity strength, balance, coordination, eccentric control, and core strength

Indications

This is a great exercise for athletes because it challenges the muscles eccentrically in a functional movement. The lunge is a difficult exercise on its own, but with the addition of the spring resistance in both directions, it is even more challenging. Not only does it emphasize eccentric quad strength and control, but it also works the glutes, hamstrings, abdominals, and lats. Balance and coordination are also challenged, and it is easy to adjust the difficulty level to make it appropriate for different objectives and levels.

Precautions or Contraindications

Non–weight-bearing status

Resistance

Light to medium (two yellow leg springs attached to the crossbar approximately half to three quarters of the way up the poles, depending on client height and strength)

Instructions

Stand between the springs of the RUB at the end of the Cadillac, facing away from it, hands holding the RUB shoulder-width apart. Separate the feet into a wide lunge stance, letting the RUB elevate to approximately 120 degrees of shoulder flexion. There should be slight tension in the springs (see photo *a*). Exhale and, keeping the torso upright, bend the knees into a lunge position and pull the RUB down to shoulder height (see photo *b*). Inhale and resist the pull of the springs to return to the starting position.

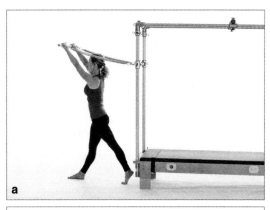

a

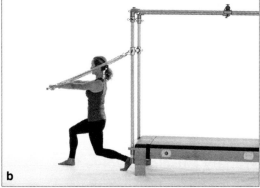

b

Progression

To increase the challenge, move the crossbar higher up the poles to create more resistance.

Technique Tips

1. Keep the front knee directly over the ankle on the down phase of the lunge, not in front of it or over the toes.
2. Ensure that the kneecap tracks directly over the second and third toes.
3. Keep the torso upright and the back straight. Do not lean forward over the front knee.
4. Posteriorly tilt the pelvis to prevent hyperlordosis and ensure activation of the glutes.
5. The back knee should almost touch the floor on the down phase of the lunge.
6. On the up phase of the lunge, keep the core and lats engaged to prevent the springs from pulling the lumbar spine into hyperextension.

STANDING ARM WORK

STANDING CHEST EXPANSION

Primary Muscles Involved

Latissimus dorsi and posterior deltoids

Objectives

Shoulder extensor strength, trunk stabilization, core control, balance, and improved posture

Indications

This exercise is essentially the same as chest expansion on the reformer (p. 128) but performed in a standing position. This makes it an excellent choice when working with patients whose conditions call for weight-bearing exercises, such as osteoporosis or poor balance or proprioception. Besides developing shoulder and arm strength, flexibility, and control, it demands upright trunk posture, good overall alignment, and core control in a functional, upright position.

Precautions or Contraindications

Non–weight-bearing status

Resistance

Medium (two yellow leg springs positioned at shoulder height or slightly above)

Instructions

Stand upright facing the RUB end of the Cadillac with the arms straight and close to the sides of the body. Hold the handles with the palms facing back, the arms slightly forward of the trunk and with slight tension on the springs.

Inhale to set the core and spread wide across the collar bones, drawing the shoulder blades down and back (see photo a). Exhale and pull the arms back as far as possible without losing the upright alignment of the trunk (see photo b). Inhale to return to the starting position.

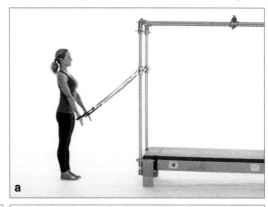

a

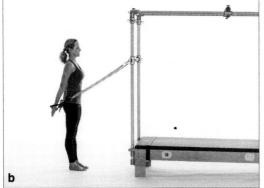

b

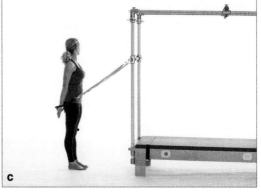

c

Variations

To improve cervical spine mobility and teach dissociation of head from trunk, add rotation of the head. When the springs are pulled back, hold the position and rotate the head slowly to the left (see photo *c*), to the right, and back to center. Return the springs to the starting position. Alternate the direction the head turns to first with each repetition. This is very effective for those who tend to tense the upper trapezius and levator scapulae muscles whenever an upper body exercise is executed (or even mentioned). Rotation of the head while the arms are engaged demonstrates the ability to achieve simultaneous upper back muscle activation and neck relaxation.

Progression

To increase the challenge, perform the exercise standing farther away from the Cadillac, balancing on one leg, or standing on an unstable surface such as a rotating disk or balance pad.

Technique Tips

1. Lengthen the arms, reaching the fingertips toward the floor.
2. Consciously pull the arms back behind the torso and resist the pull of the springs when returning the arms forward, rather than swinging the arms back and forth.

STANDING HUG A TREE

Primary Muscles Involved

Pectoralis major

Objective

Horizontal adductor strength, pec stretch, trunk and scapular stabilization, and improved posture, balance, and core control

Indications

As with all of the exercises in the standing arm work series, this is an excellent choice when working with patients whose conditions call for weight-bearing exercises, such as osteoporosis or poor balance or proprioception. Besides developing shoulder and arm strength, flexibility, and control, it demands upright trunk posture, good overall alignment, and core control in a functional, upright position.

Precautions or Contraindications

Non–weight-bearing status

Resistance

Medium (two yellow leg springs positioned at shoulder height or slightly above)

Instructions

Stand upright with the feet hip-width apart, facing away from RUB end of Cadillac. Hold the handles in a *T* position with soft elbows and palms facing forward. Engage the abdominals and lean the trunk forward slightly against the resistance of the springs (see photo *a*). Exhale and draw the arms toward each other until they are parallel, hands in line with shoulders (see photo *b*), then inhale and return to the starting position.

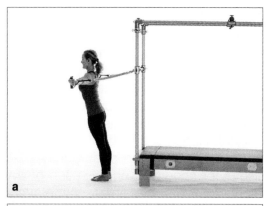

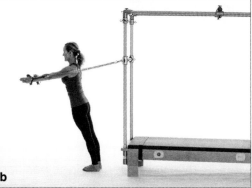

Progression

To increase the challenge, perform standing farther away from the Cadillac, move the feet closer together, balance on one leg or stand on an unstable surface such as a rotating disk or balance pad.

Technique Tips

1. Maintain good posture and alignment by keeping the abdominals engaged throughout the exercise and leaning slightly forward against the springs.
2. Keep the arms elongated but the elbows soft, while reaching out through the fingertips.
3. Lead with the pinky finger so the shoulders are in slight external rotation.
4. Maintain proper scapular stabilization by drawing the shoulder blades down and back.

STANDING ARM CIRCLES

Primary Muscles Involved

Shoulder extensors and horizontal adductors

Objectives

Shoulder mobility, shoulder strength and control, trunk and scapular stabilization, and improved posture, balance, and core control

Indications

As with all of the exercises in the standing arm work series, this is an excellent choice when working with patients whose conditions call for weight-bearing exercises such as osteoporosis or poor balance or proprioception. Besides developing shoulder and arm strength, flexibility, and control, it demands upright trunk posture, good overall alignment, and core control in a functional, upright position. Because this exercise goes into the overhead position, it is very challenging for shoulder strength and scapular stability. It also helps increase or maintain shoulder elevation range of motion. It is especially useful for shoulder rehabilitation of overhead sport athletes such as swimmers, volleyball players, tennis players, and water polo players. It is also a huge challenge to core control and trunk stabilization. For nonathletes, it is still very useful since we all need to be able to reach and lift overhead with a stabilized scapula.

Precautions or Contraindications

Non–weight-bearing status, shoulder impingement syndrome, rotator cuff tendinitis or tear, early to mid-stage status post-op rotator cuff repair, or pain with overhead motion

Resistance

Medium (two yellow leg springs positioned at shoulder height or slightly above)

Instructions

Stand upright facing away from the RUB end of the Cadillac with feet hip-width apart. Hold the handles in a *T* position with soft elbows and palms facing forward. Engage the abdominals and lean the trunk forward slightly against the resistance of the springs (see photo *a*).

Standing Up Circles

Exhale and draw the arms toward each other until they are parallel, hands in line with the shoulders (see photo *b*). Inhale and rotate the palms to face down and lift the arms overhead (see photo *c*). Circle the arms out to the sides and return to the starting position (see photo *d*). Repeat 5 to 10 times and then reverse direction.

Progression

To increase the challenge, perform the exercise standing farther away from the Cadillac, move the feet closer together, balance on one leg, or stand on an unstable surface such as a rotating disk or balance pad.

Technique Tips

1. Keep the movement smooth as in supine arm circles on the reformer (p. 99) and kneeling arm circles on the reformer (p. 134).
2. Do not let the hands go behind the torso.

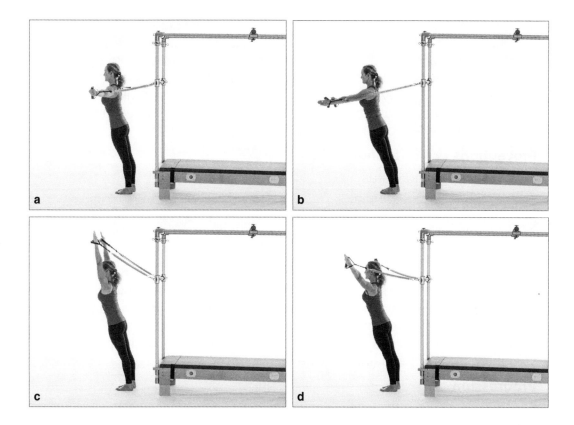

3. Keep the core engaged and maintain the upright position of the trunk.
4. Keep the scapulae depressed so the shoulders do not rise up toward the ears as the arms are elevated.

STANDING BICEPS

Primary Muscles Involved

Biceps

Objectives

Elbow flexor strength, scapular adductor strength, anterior shoulder and pec stretch, scapular and trunk stabilization, improved posture, balance, and core control

Indications

As with all of the exercises in the standing arm work series, this is an excellent choice when working with patients whose conditions call for weight-bearing exercises such as osteoporosis or poor balance or proprioception. Besides developing shoulder and arm strength, flexibility, and control, it demands upright trunk posture, good overall alignment, and core control in a functional, upright position. This exercise gives us an excellent alternative position in which to work the biceps—one that counteracts the tendency to round the shoulders forward and use the pecs. With the arms behind the back, the chest is open, the upper body is not rounded forward, and the scapular adductors are working. Scapular and trunk stabilization are also challenged in this position and by the direction of resistance.

Precautions or Contraindications

Non–weight-bearing status

Resistance

Medium (two yellow leg springs positioned at shoulder height or slightly above)

Instructions

Stand upright facing away from the RUB end of the Cadillac with the feet hip-width apart. Hold the handles and lean slightly forward, reaching the arms behind the body parallel to each other. Draw back through the elbows as the collar bones lift (see photo a). Exhale and bend the elbows, keeping the arms still and elbows at a consistent height (see photo b), and then inhale to straighten the arms and return to the starting position.

Progression

To increase the challenge, perform the exercise standing farther away from the Cadillac, move the feet closer together, balance on one leg, or stand on an unstable surface such as a rotating disk or balance pad.

Technique Tips

1. Keep the elbows and upper arms still and parallel to each other, with the shoulders in extension.
2. Spread across the collar bones and keep the scapular adductors engaged to keep the shoulder heads from falling or rounding forward.
3. Keep the abdominals engaged and avoid thrusting the ribs forward.

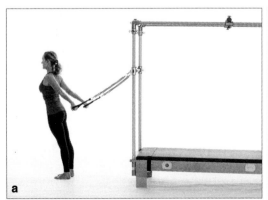
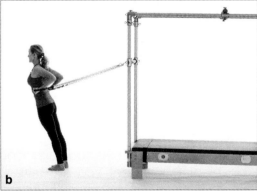

a

b

8

Wunda Chair Exercises

The wunda or combo chair lends itself to many effective core and upper extremity exercises, but I use it most for rehab and prehab of patients with hip and knee injuries or balance issues. It is a great tool for progressing weight-bearing status, from the supine zero gravity position on the reformer to unsupported sitting and eventually standing exercises on the chair. The chair is a key piece of equipment to have in a Pilates-based rehab center because it is versatile, lightweight, relatively inexpensive, doesn't take up too much space, and allows for many weight-bearing functional exercises.

As with the reformer and Cadillac, the resistance is provided by springs. However, the resistance on the wunda or combo chair is a bit more difficult to standardize due to differences among manufacturers in both the resistance provided by individual springs and varying adjustment systems. I recommend experimenting to ensure that the spring system on your particular chair is thoroughly understood before prescribing exercises to patients. The following guidelines can be used:

Lightest setting = one light spring (usually white) at the lowest position on one pedal

Heaviest setting = two heavy springs (usually black) at the highest position on each pedal

The exercise instructions are written in a voice such that a professional can instruct his or her patient or client, and such that the directions can be followed by the practitioner him or herself. I recommend that anyone who does not have experience with Pilates works with a certified instructor to practice the exercises- both in the role of the client and of the teacher- before applying them in a rehabilitation practice. This is essential in being able to provide a safe and effective exercise program.

Pelvic Curl

Primary Muscles Involved

Abdominals and hamstrings

Objectives

Mobilization of the spine and pelvic region, spinal articulation, hamstring strength and control, pelvic lumbar stabilization, and recruitment and cocontraction of the core muscles

Indications

This is another version of the pelvic curl on the mat (p. 57) with the added benefit of challenging the hamstrings. It is a great exercise for those with general stiffness or arthritis of the spine, a weak or inhibited core, or tightness of back extensors or hip flexors. It is a great way to begin a Pilates session as it promotes relaxation and the mind–body connection, and it gets the spine moving and primed for more challenging exercises.

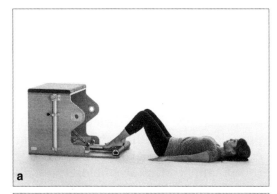

Precautions or Contraindications

Acute lumbar disk pathology or osteoporosis (due to the deep spinal flexion)

Resistance

Extra light to light

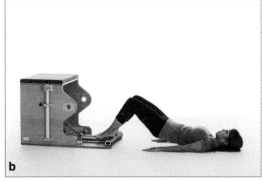

Instructions

Lie supine on the floor in a neutral pelvis position with the knees bent and the heels on the pedal. The arms should be relaxed at the sides with the palms down. Inhale to press the pedal down to the floor (see photo a). Exhale to engage the core, then curl the pelvis and spine off the floor one vertebra at a time, holding the pedal down (see photo b). Inhale and pause at the top of the available range of motion. Ideally there is a diagonal line of energy from the shoulders through the hips to the knees (see photo c). Exhale and roll

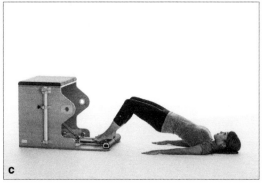

down to the starting the position one vertebra at a time, again keeping the pedal down.

Variations

1. For patients with disk pathologies, omit the deep lumbar flexion and maintain the spine and pelvis in a neutral position as it is lifted.
2. Place a ball between the knees to promote more adductor engagement.
3. Reach the arms overhead as the pelvis lifts to elicit more upper spine control.

Technique Tips

1. Think of pulling the heels toward the tailbone to keep the hamstrings engaged and the pelvis posteriorly tilted.
2. Keep the neck and shoulders relaxed.
3. Maximize lumbar flexion as the spine lifts off the mat by pulling the pubic bone towards the chin (posteriorly tilting the pelvis).
4. Visualize the lowering of the spine like a Slinky spring toy going down steps, deliberately placing one vertebra at a time. This will help to achieve maximum articulation and spinal mobility.

HAMSTRING CURL

Primary Muscles Involved

Hamstrings

Objectives

Hamstring strength and control and lumbo-pelvic stabilization

Indications

Most hamstring curl exercises are done in the prone position, which puts the lumbar spine in danger of being pulled into hyperextension. This setup on the wunda chair provides a way to isolate the hamstrings in a stable and comfortable position for the spine, making it useful for people suffering from acute lumbar or sacroiliac joint pain, stenosis, or spondylolisthesis. It can also be performed unilaterally, which is great for muscular imbalances or postsurgical strengthening.

Precautions or Contraindications

Acute hamstring injury

Resistance

Light

Instructions

Lie supine on the floor in a neutral position with the knees flexed at approximately 90 degrees and the heels on the pedals of the wunda chair. The legs should be parallel and the arms resting by the sides (see photo *a*). Exhale to bend the knees and pull the pedal halfway down (see photo *b*). Inhale and, with control, slowly return the pedal to the starting position by extending the knees.

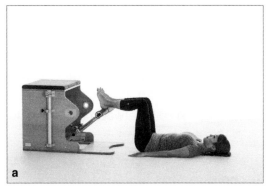

Progression

Perform the exercise unilaterally, with the opposite leg held in the tabletop position.

Technique Tips

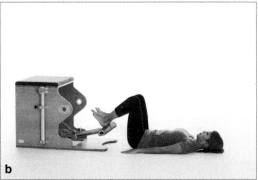

1. Maintain a neutral pelvis position (or appropriate pelvic position for the specific condition) throughout the series.
2. Visualize a rubber band connecting each heel to the opposite sit bone. As the knees bend, pull the heels towards the sit bones, shortening the rubber band. As the knees straighten, the band stretches, creating a strong pull between the heel and sit bones. Resist the movement as if trying to keep knees bent. This internal resistance increases the work in the muscles, maximizing the eccentric contraction.
3. Do not take the pedal all the way to the floor, as this causes the pelvis to go into an anterior tilt and lose connection with the hamstrings.

MODIFIED SWAN ON FLOOR

Primary Muscles Involved

Middle and lower trapezius

Objectives

To retrain coactivation of the upper core (deep neck flexors, lower trapezius, and serratus anterior), back extensor strength, middle and lower trapezius strength and control, and scapular stabilization and movement

Indications

This is a wonderful exercise for those with very stiff thoracic spines or scapulae that do not move. So many people (especially those who tend to stress, spend many hours at the computer, or who are overhead sport athletes) overwork their upper trapezius but have difficulty engaging or even finding the middle and lower trapezius. The scapulae then become hypomobile or stiff. The lower trapezius is one of the most commonly weak or inhibited muscles of the scapulothoracic joint that may lead to abnormal movement. The position of the body and the pedal on the wunda chair, as well as the direction of resistance, works very well in recruiting the lower trapezius and providing tangible feedback. Pressing into the pedal activates the serratus anterior. An added benefit is that the body is held in trunk extension, so it is wonderful for strengthening the back body and improving posture.

Precautions or Contraindications

Contraindications include acute shoulder impingement syndrome, spondylolisthesis, and acute neck or lower back pain. Use caution with cervical or lumbar stenosis.

Resistance

Extra light to light

Instructions

Lie prone on the floor in a sphinx positon (propped up on the elbows). Instructor pushes the pedal down so that the patient can place the hands on the pedal without stressing the neck or shoulder (see photo *a*). The patient then lifts into spinal extension, placing both wrists on the pedal. Engage the core muscles, perhaps slightly posteriorly tilting the pelvis to protect the lumbar spine (see photo *b*). Inhale and pull the pedal toward the body, pressing it down slightly by drawing the shoulder blades down and back toward the pelvis (see photo *c*). Exhale to slowly return the pedal to the starting position. Repeat for 10 to 20 repetitions of scapular depression and elevation while maintaining back exten-

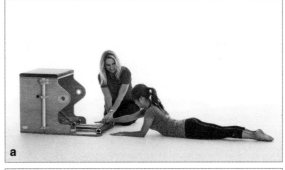

a

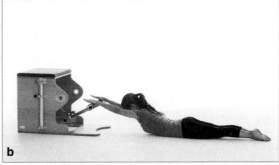

b

sion. Upon completion of the last repetition, instructor holds the pedal still so that the patient can return to the sphinx position safely (see photo *d*).

Variations

If there are no neck or shoulder issues, the exercise can be performed the classical way in which there is no assistance from the instructor. From a prone position on the floor, reach the hands to the pedal with the forehead resting on the floor (see photo *e*). Inhale to extend the back while pressing the pedal down (see photo *f*). Exhale and lower the body back to the floor as the pedal rises back to the starting position. This version emphasizes back extensor strength and range of motion rather than scapular mobility and lower trapezius strength and control.

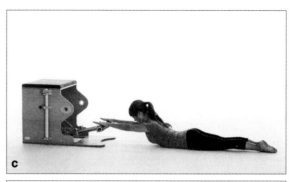

c

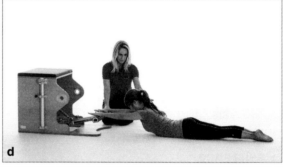

d

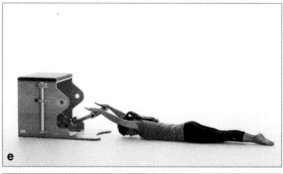

e

Technique Tips

1. Avoid jutting the chin forward by maintaining the chin nod throughout the exercise.

2. Rather than thinking of lifting the head, think of reaching the crown of the head away from the tailbone, elongating through the neck.

3. Keep the abdominals engaged throughout the exercise.

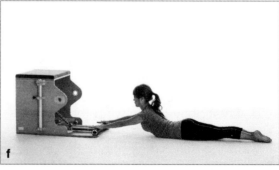

f

4. Visualize the scapulae sliding down the back toward the hips.

5. In the scapular elevation phase, do not allow the shoulders to move up toward the ears (minimize upper trapezius activity).

6. Tactile cueing at the inferior borders of the scapulae is very effective in this position.

SINGLE-ARM PUSH-UP

*A variation of an original exercise taught by Rael Isacowitz in the BASI Mentor Program (Isacowitz 2018).

Primary Muscles Involved

Pectoralis major and minor

Objectives

Shoulder horizontal adduction strength, scapular stabilization, lumbo-pelvic stabilization, and recruitment and cocontraction of the core muscles

Indications

This is another example of a full-body integration exercise. Exercises in this block rely on integration of the whole body for performance, rather than a single region. Full-body integration exercises are closed chain, which makes them very functional and thus crucial in injury rehab and for athletes. This push-up series is very challenging to the entire body, but a simple change of lower body position makes it appropriate for almost anyone. It is done in a specific way to emphasize activation and strength of the pectoralis minor (rather than the pectoralis major, which is the focus of traditional push-ups), an important yet often forgotten scapular stabilizer.

Precautions or Contraindications

Knee pads or a thick mat for patients with sensitive knees

Resistance

Use medium to heavy resistance. The resistance can be very tricky for this exercise; it needs to be light enough to be able to isolate the pectoralis minor in pushing the pedal down, but heavy enough to support the body in a unilateral plank position.

Instructions

Get in a quadruped position on the floor to the side of the chair, with the spine in a neutral position, the knees directly under the hips and the supporting hand directly under that shoulder. Place the opposite elbow and forearm on the pedal (see photo a). Engage the core muscles and set the scapula by drawing it down and back. Press the supporting hand into the floor to recruit the serratus anterior. Exhale and pull the pedal in toward the body with the elbow (horizontal adduction). When it is impossible to push any farther with the elbow, let the elbow float off but continue pressing the pedal to the floor with the hand (see photo b). Inhale and, with control, allow the pedal to return slowly to the elbow, and then slowly abduct the arm back to the starting positon.

Progression

1. Perform the exercise in half quadruped position (see photo c).
2. Perform the exercise in a full plank position, with the knees off the floor (see photo d).

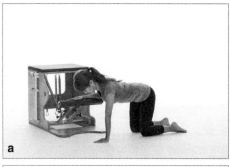
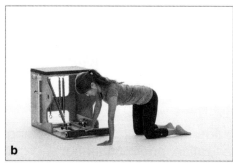
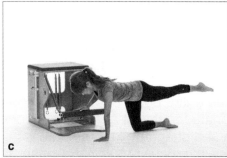
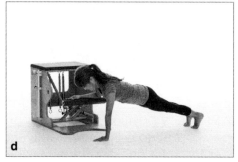

3. For even less stability and thus more core challenge, move the body back so that the elbow is not touching the pedal at the start of the exercise.

Technique Tips

1. Keep the core muscles engaged throughout the exercise.
2. The pushing hand will be slightly forward of the supporting hand when both are in the down position.
3. Avoid the tendency to simply push the pedal down (working more triceps and pectoralis major). Instead, emphasize pulling the elbow in toward the body as much as possible.

REVERSE SHRUGS

Primary Muscles Involved

Middle and lower trapezius

Objectives

Scapular depressor strength, trunk stabilization, and improved posture

Indications

Overhead sport athletes, people with occupations such as painter or hairdresser, and even those who spend many hours at the computer tend to have an overdeveloped and tight upper trapezius but difficulty engaging or even finding the middle and lower trapezius. As opposed to traditional shrugs, which strengthen the upper trapezius, these shrugs strengthen the middle and lower trapezius, which are so important in ensuring proper scapulothoracic movement and thus preventing neck and shoulder injuries.

Precautions or Contraindications

None

Resistance

Medium

Instructions

Sit on a small box on the floor facing away from the chair with the legs together, knees bent, and feet flat on the floor. Place the hands on the pedal with the fingers facing the body. Press the pedal down with the arms. Draw the shoulders back (see photo *a*). Inhale to let the pedal and shoulders rise (see photo *b*). Exhale and press the pedal down.

Variations

Taller clients or those with tight hip flexors can sit on a larger box.

Progression

To increase core stabilization challenge, place a spinning disc or balance cushion on top of the box, or sit on a foam roll instead of the box.

Technique Tips

1. There is a tendency to lean back into the pedals. Avoid this by cocontracting the abdominals and back extensors and keeping the torso upright and centered on the box.
2. Keep the scapular adductors engaged throughout the exercise (draw the shoulder blades together).
3. Spread wide across the collar bones and avoid letting the shoulders round forward.
4. When elevating, the shoulders should raise straight up toward the ears rather than forward or back.

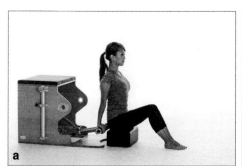 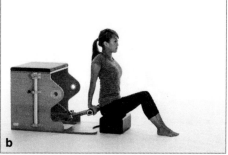

TRICEPS PRESS SIT

Primary Muscles Involved

Triceps

Objectives

Elbow extensor strength, scapular stabilization, trunk stabilization, and improved posture

Indications

This exercise provides a simple way to work the triceps that also challenges core strength and emphasizes upright posture. Besides the elbow extensors, scapular retractors and depressors are also recruited.

Precautions or Contraindications

Acute shoulder impingement syndrome

Resistance

Medium

Instructions

Sit on a small box on the floor facing away from the chair with the legs together, knees bent, and feet flat on floor. Place the hands on the pedal with the fingers facing the body, and the elbows bent and pulling towards each other (see photo a). Exhale and press the pedal down by straightening the elbows (see photo b). Inhale and bend the elbows to return the pedal to the starting position.

Variations

As indicated for the reverse shrugs, taller people or those with tight hip flexors can sit on a larger box.

Progression

Similar to the reverse shrugs, to increase core stabilization challenge, have the patient sit on a foam roll instead of the box or place a spinning disc on top of the box.

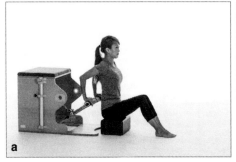
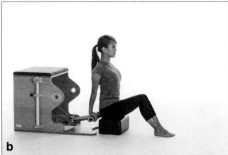

Technique Tips

1. Keep the trunk upright and the core muscles engaged. Do not lean back.
2. Keep the middle and lower trapezius engaged by drawing the shoulder blades down and back throughout the exercise.
3. Spread wide across the collar bones and avoid letting the shoulders roll forward.
4. Keep the elbows parallel to each other.
5. Visualize the scapulae gliding down the back and the body lifting off the box as the pedal is pressed down.

PRONE TRICEPS

Primary Muscles Involved

Triceps

Objectives

Elbow extensor strength, trunk extensor strength, and scapular and trunk stabilization

Indications

This is another great way to strengthen the triceps, with the added benefit of challenging core strength and control. The movement is the same as that of a push-up but in a non–weight-bearing position, making it a great way to teach proper push-up form. Even those lacking sufficient core strength to hold the body in a plank position can do this "push-up" without risk of collapsing in the lumbo-pelvic region.

Precautions or Contraindications

Spondylolisthesis

Resistance

Medium

Instructions

Lie prone over the chair with the legs straight and together. Place the hands on the pedal, with the arms extended and the shoulders aligned over the wrists. The fingers face straight forward and the elbows pull in toward each other to keep them parallel. Engage the core and slightly tuck the tailbone to protect the lumbar spine from excessive extension (see photo a). Inhale and bend the elbows (see photo b), then exhale and straighten the elbows.

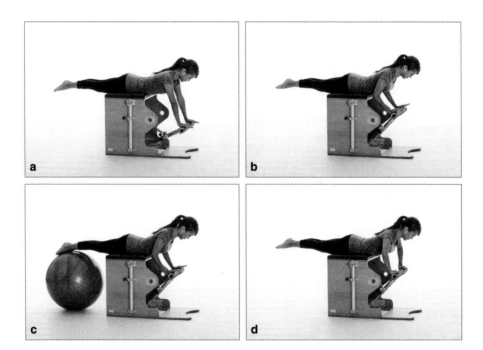

Variations

1. To make the exercise easier, place a large physio ball under the feet to support the lower body (see photo c).
2. To emphasize pec strength or prepare for pec push-ups, widen the hands, turn the fingers in, and rotate the elbows out (see photo d).

Progression

Perform the exercise unilaterally, with one arm reaching out to the side, palm down. This increases the challenge to both arm strength and core stabilization.

Technique Tips

1. Keep the body parallel to the floor and completely still.
2. Keep the abdominals and back extensors cocontracted throughout the exercise.
3. Keep the head in line with the spine.
4. In the unilateral version, do not let the body rotate. The body should be in a straight line and look as if both arms were pushing the pedal.

BASIC SWAN (BACK EXTENSION)

Primary Muscles Involved

Back extensors

Objectives

Back extensor strength, scapular stabilization, abdominal control, and improved posture

Indications

This is a wonderful exercise after a back injury because it provides neuromuscular reeducation to the extensors. The spring tension can be regulated to provide assistance in the beginning and later can be decreased gradually as the client heals and the back muscles become stronger. It is also a great way to teach proper cocontraction of the core muscles during back extension, as the abdominals must be recruited to prevent overarching in the lumbar area. It is a great postural exercise, as the pedals encourage shoulder opening as the trunk extends.

Precautions or Contraindications

Spondylolisthesis, stenosis, or acute back injury or pain

Resistance

Light or medium to assist in range of motion only; lighter to challenge extensor strength

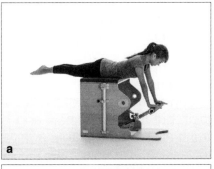

Instructions

Lie prone over the chair with the legs straight and together and the trunk parallel to the floor. Place the hands on the pedal with the shoulders aligned over the wrists and the arms straight. Engage the abdominals (see photo a). Inhale and extend the spine as the pedal rises (see photo b). Exhale slowly, and with control, return to the starting position.

Variations

To make the exercise easier, place a large physio ball under the feet to support the lower body (see prone triceps photo c, p. 206).

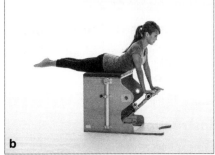

Progression

Perform the exercise unilaterally. Begin in the same position but with one arm reaching straight out to the side. Inhale and extend the spine to lift the pedal up, keeping the opposite arm completely still, and then exhale and lower to the starting position.

Technique Tips

1. Begin the articulation of the spine with the head (as long as there are no neck issues). The idea is to create a gentle arc of the entire spine rather than hinging at the lumbar spine which results in severe hyperextension in this region.
2. Keep the abdominals engaged throughout.
3. Keep the adductors engaged.
4. In the single-arm version, do not allow any rotation or lateral flexion of the spine when lifting and lowering.

TORSO PRESS SIT

Primary Muscles Involved

Abdominals and back extensors

Objectives

Abdominal and back extensor strength, core stabilization and control, shoulder and chest stretch, hip flexor control, and improved posture

Indications

This is a very difficult exercise to do correctly, but a great way to challenge strength and control of the entire body. The movement takes place at the hip joint, but the abdominals and back extensors must cocontract to keep the trunk aligned and stable against gravity. It is also a great exercise for desk jockeys, as it counteracts poor sitting posture by encouraging back extension and shoulder opening.

Precautions or Contraindications

Spondylolisthesis, acute back pain, or hip flexor injury

Resistance

Extra light to light

Instructions

Sit on the chair with the back facing the pedal. Place the hands on the pedal with the fingers facing away from the body, shoulders aligned over the hands with straight arms. Extend the legs out parallel to the floor and hold the trunk in a diagonal line (see photo a). Inhale to lower the body and the pedal toward the floor until the body is parallel to the floor (see photo b). Exhale to return to the starting position.

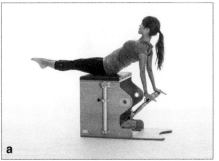 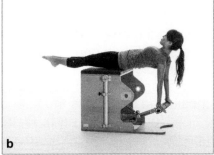

a   b

Variations

Place a large physio ball or box under the feet to support the legs and decrease the load on the hip flexors.

Technique Tips

1. Maintain cocontraction of the abdominals and back extensors throughout the exercise.
2. The head should be aligned with the spine throughout the movement, and the deep neck flexors should be gently engaged.
3. The legs should remain completely still and parallel to the floor.
4. Visualize the body lengthening, reaching the head and feet away from each other to grow as tall as possible.

PIRIFORMIS STRETCH

Primary Muscles Involved

Piriformis

Objectives

To stretch the piriformis and Achilles tendon

Indications

This provides a nice alternative to the pigeon stretch often done in yoga. In this version, there is less pressure on the knee as the position supports more body weight than when done on the floor. Added bonuses are an Achilles tendon stretch of the opposite leg and a gentle release of the trunk muscles.

Precautions or Contraindications

Contraindications include lumbar disk pathology, osteoporosis, or acute knee injury. Use caution with post-op total hip replacement patients.

Resistance

Light

Instructions

Stand behind the chair facing the seat on the spring side. Place one leg on the seat in a comfortable pigeon position (hip in external rotation). Reach straight back with the opposite leg and press the heel down on the floor (or a box or pad). Place the hands on the pedal (see photo *a*). Exhale to press the pedal to the floor, completely relaxing the body over the chair (see photo *b*). Hold the stretch and breathe for 30 seconds to 1 minute.

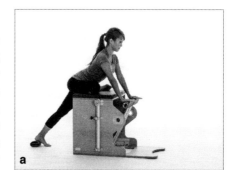

a

Variations

Before or after holding the stretch, the body can be lifted in and out of the stretch position slowly. Inhale as the pedal is lifted and exhale to press the pedal to the floor.

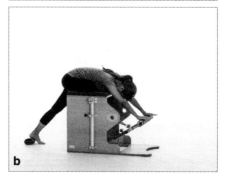

b

Technique Tips

1. For more of a stretch, place the foot closer to the top of the seat with the shin parallel to it. People with tighter muscles will need to have the foot lower on the seat, closer to the pelvis.

2. In order to get the Achilles stretch, it is important that the foot is flat against a surface (the floor for taller people, on a box or pad for shorter people).

CALF PRESS

Primary Muscles Involved

Foot plantar flexors (soleus, tibialis posterior, peroneus [fibularis] longus and brevis, plantaris, flexor digitorum longus, and flexor hallucis longus)

Objectives

Plantar flexor strength and calf and hip flexor stretch

Indications

This is a simple way to isolate the one-joint plantar flexors in a functional position. Range of motion, strength, and flexibility of the calf are all addressed with this movement. The position is very good for teaching proper foot alignment. Added benefits are the hip flexor stretch felt on the standing leg and the core stability needed to maintain the position in the more advanced versions. It can also be used to challenge balance.

Precautions or Contraindications

Non–weight-bearing status

Resistance

Medium to heavy

Instructions

Stand on the floor facing the pedal of the chair and place the toes of one foot on the pedal and the part of the knee just below the kneecap into the front edge of the seat. A pad can be placed between the knee and the seat for increased comfort. The back leg is straight with the heel on the floor and the toes facing straight forward. Place the hands on the sides of the seat (see photo a). Exhale to press the pedal down by plantar flexing the foot (see photo b). Inhale to dorsi flex the foot and return the pedal to the starting position.

Variations

The arms can reach out to the sides or behind the head to increase the balance challenge.

Progression

Add upper body movement or resistance such as diagonal pulls with a resistance band to challenge balance and coordination (see photo c).

Technique Tips

1. Maintain the hips square and the body in a long diagonal line from the back heel to the head.
2. Emphasize control of the pedal through the full range of motion.

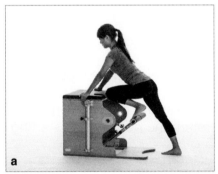

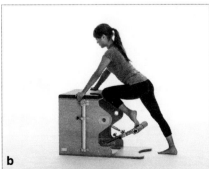

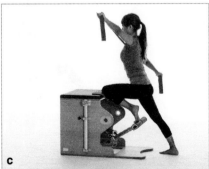

3. Maintain abdominal engagement.
4. If no stretch is felt in the back leg (Achilles and hip flexor), step back farther and make sure that the toes are facing straight forward (not rotated out to the side).

STANDING LEG PRESS

Primary Muscles Involved
Hamstrings and gluteus medius

Objectives
Improved balance, hip extensor strength, lateral hip stability, and improved upright posture

Indications
This is a great exercise to challenge balance, proprioception, lateral hip stability, and lower extremity eccentric control. It is a very functional movement, similar to walking up stairs, so it is very useful in neuromuscular reeducation after a period of non–weight bearing due to a knee, hip, or ankle injury or surgery. It is also a great choice for clients with osteoporosis.

Precautions or Contraindications
Non–weight-bearing status

Resistance
Light to medium

Instructions
Stand on the floor facing the chair with the toes of one foot on the pedal. Stand up tall, with the abdominals engaged and the arms reaching out to a *T* position (see photo *a*). Exhale to press the pedal down to the base of the chair (see photo *b*) and inhale to return the pedal to the starting position with control.

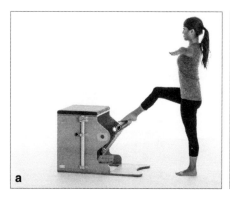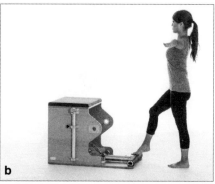

Variations

1. Traditionally this exercise is done standing back approximately 12 to 24 inches (30.5 to 61 cm) from the chair, with the foot in plantar flexion on the pedal. I find this position is too difficult for my older clients to maintain balance, so I let them stand as close to the chair as possible and place the middle of the foot flat on the pedal. If they are unable to balance on one leg without assistance, I either provide manual assistance for them or let them hold a gondola pole.

2. To increase activation of the glutes and challenge balance in a different plane, turn sideways to the chair so that the hip is in external rotation when pressing the pedal down.

Progression

Stand on a spinning disc, half foam roll, or balance pad.

Technique Tips

1. Stand completely upright; do not lean forward or back.
2. Initiate the movement from the hip extensors rather than the knee extensors.

FORWARD LUNGE

Primary Muscles Involved

Hamstrings, gluteus medius, and quadriceps

Objectives

Hip extensor, hip abductor, and knee extensor strength and improved balance

Indications

This is one of my favorite exercises for athletes, especially for any sport that involves running or jumping. It is very challenging! To do it correctly takes excellent balance, strength, control, muscle patterning, and lumbo-pelvic stability. Correct execution requires initiating the lift-off with the hip extensors, lateral stability as the foot comes off the pedal, and quadriceps strength and control for terminal knee extension at the top.

Precautions or Contraindications

Non–weight-bearing status, lower extremity osteoarthritis, knee pathologies that are aggravated by weight-bearing deep knee bends (meniscus tear, patellofemoral pain syndrome, or patellar tendinitis)

Resistance

Heavy; less resistance is more challenging

Instructions

Stand with one foot on the chair with the knee aligned over the second and third toes, and the other foot in plantar flexion pressing the pedal to the floor. Stand upright with the hips directly over the pedal and the core muscles engaged. Reach the arms out to a *T* position or clasp them behind the head (see photo *a*). Exhale to press the heel of the front foot into the seat and straighten that leg as the pedal rises (see photo *b*). Continue straightening the leg to full knee extension as the foot lifts off the pedal and taps the back edge of the seat (see photo *c*). Inhale to lower with control until the thigh is parallel to the floor (see photo *d*). Repeat 8 to 10 times before lowering the pedal all the way to the floor, or hold the last repetition and flow into the next exercise (backward step-down, p. 216).

Variations

As mentioned, this is a very difficult exercise so there are a few ways to modify it.

1. The handles on the chair can be used to teach the mechanics of this exercise, or they can be used in the beginning for severe weakness (see

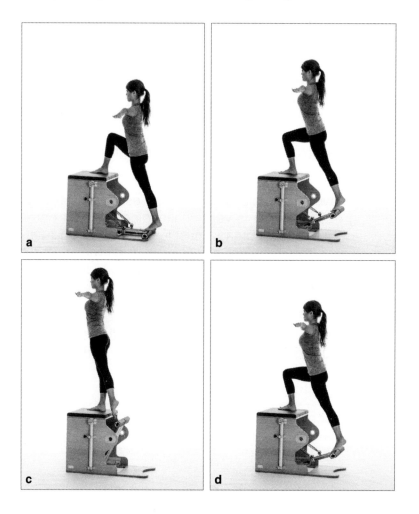

photo *e*). However, the tendency is to lean forward onto the handles, which changes the muscle focus. It is best to wean off of this version as soon as possible so that the correct form and muscle recruitment can be learned.

2. Place the wunda chair at the edge of the Cadillac so that the upright poles can be used for balance.

3. Use a gondola pole to assist with balance.

4. For knee pathologies in which weight-bearing deep knee flexion is contraindicated but terminal knee extension, quadriceps, and gluteus medius strengthening is desired, a box can be placed at the base of the wunda chair to limit the amount of knee flexion. Have the patient mount the chair as if climbing a staircase so that it is not necessary to load the knee in deep flexion (see photos *f* and *g*).

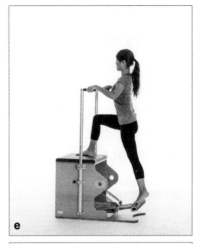

Progression

A balance pad or spinning disc can be placed on the seat of the chair to further challenge balance and proprioception.

Technique Tips

1. Placing a mirror in front of the client is very useful in teaching proper technique and lower extremity alignment for this exercise.

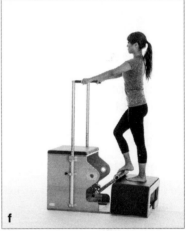

2. The muscles should be activated sequentially: first, hip extensors, then hip abductors, and finally knee extensors.

3. To get the full benefit of the exercise, it is very important to emphasize terminal knee extension in single-leg stance at the top. This ensures activation of the vastus medius oblique. Draw the kneecap up to achieve this.

4. It should feel as if the body is levitating straight up toward the ceiling. Press into the front heel as the body rises up and down and avoid leaning forward.

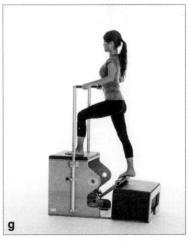

5. The pelvis should remain stable and level throughout. The tendency is for it to drop, especially as the foot lifts off the pedal. A lot of gluteus medius activation is required at that point to avoid this.

6. The knee should remain aligned directly over the second and third toes throughout the exercise.

BACKWARD STEP-DOWN

Primary Muscles Involved

Gluteal muscles, hamstrings, and quadriceps

Objectives

Hip extensor and abductor strength, isometric quadriceps strength and control, and improved balance

Indications

This is another great exercise for athletes because it strengthens the hip abductors in a functional position, challenges knee stability and control, and encourages proper patellofemoral alignment. Of course, the core muscles are also working to maintain lumbo-pelvic stabilization. The focus is on the hip abductors, especially the gluteus medius, which is often weak compared to the overused quadriceps and hamstrings. This is very common in athletes whose activities are sagittal plane dominant (running, cycling, flutter kick swimming). This muscle imbalance can be a contributing factor in pathologies such as patellofemoral pain syndrome, iliotibial band syndrome, and patellar tendinopathy. As with the forward lunge, to do it correctly takes excellent balance, strength, control, muscle patterning, and lumbo-pelvic stability.

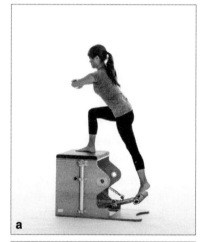

a

Precautions or Contraindications

Non–weight-bearing status or lower extremity osteoarthritis

Resistance

Use medium to heavy resistance. As with the forward lunge, less resistance is more challenging.

Instructions

Stand with one foot on the seat of the chair with the knee aligned over second and third toes and the other foot in plantar flexion on the pedal. Lean the body slightly forward with all of the weight on the front leg and bring the thigh parallel to the floor and the pedal approximately halfway up. The back should be flat on a diagonal with the abdominals engaged and the arms crossed in front of the chest (see photo *a*). Inhale to bend the back leg and exhale to straighten it (in a pumping motion) by pressing the pedal up and down (see photo *b*). The standing leg should remain completely still.

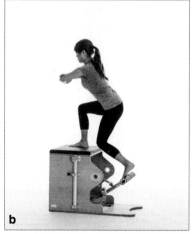

b

Note: This exercise flows well from forward lunge. Hold the last repetition of the forward lunge (see photo *d* p. 214 halfway down (thigh parallel to floor) and begin backward step-down. After the last repetition of backward step-down, finish by rising to the end position of the forward lunge, place both feet on the seat, switch legs, and repeat the sequence.

Variations

1. As with the forward lunge, the handles can be used to teach the mechanics of this exercise, or for severe weakness; see photo *e*, page 215. However, the tendency is to lean forward onto the handles, which changes the muscle focus. It is best to wean off of this version as soon as possible so that the correct form and muscle recruitment can be learned.
2. The upright poles of the Cadillac or a gondola pole can be used if needed for balance and assistance.
3. The arms can reach straight up overhead.

Progression

A balance pad or spinning disc can be placed on the seat to further challenge balance and proprioception.

Technique Tips

1. There is a tendency to move the hip of the supporting leg up and down as the pedal moves. Press into the heel of the foot on the seat and actively engage the glutes to prevent this.
2. The knee of the supporting leg should be directly over the ankle and toes. Do not allow it to move forward of the toes as this places too much pressure on the knee joint.
3. The pelvis should remain stable and level.
4. The foot on the pedal should remain in plantar flexion.

CALF PRESS IN FORWARD LUNGE

Primary Muscles Involved

Gastrocnemius

Objectives

Plantar flexor strength, gluteus medius strength, hip and knee stability and control, and improved balance

Indications

This is another great exercise for athletes because it strengthens the gastrocnemius in a functional position, challenges knee stability and control, and requires excellent balance and core stabilization. The gastrocnemius is an important knee stabilizer that is often neglected in knee rehabilitation as we are more focused on the quadriceps and hamstrings. When there is weakness or tightness in the gastrocnemius, the other muscles of the knee are forced to work harder to stabilize the patellofemoral joint, resulting in muscle imbalances and contributing to pathologies such as patellar and hamstring tendinopathies. An added benefit of this position is that it forces the gluteus medius to laterally stabilize the hip which challenges balance and thereby helps one to improve it. This exercise is another example of full body integration!

Precautions or Contraindications

Non–weight-bearing status or lower extremity osteoarthritis (due to load on the supporting leg)

Resistance

Medium

Instructions

Place one foot on the chair, with the knee aligned over the second and third toes and the other foot on the pedal, approximately three quarters of the way up. Stand upright with the hips directly over the pedal and the core muscles engaged. Reach out to a *T* position with the arms or clasp them behind the head (see photo *a*).

Exhale to plantar flex the foot on the pedal, keeping the knee fully extended and the rest of the body completely still (see photo *b*). Inhale to dorsi flex the foot, controlling the pedal as it rises.

Note: This exercise, like the backward step-down, flows well from the forward lunge (p. 213).

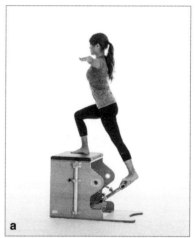

a

Variations

Arms can reach up to the ceiling, or hold a ball or magic circle to activate the upper body muscles.

Progression

A balance pad or spinning disc can be placed on the seat to further challenge balance and proprioception.

Technique Tips

1. Keep the knee of the supporting leg aligned directly over the ankle and toes. Do not allow it to move forward of the toes as this places too much pressure on the knee joint.

2. Stand up tall and keep the core muscles engaged.

3. Keep the pelvis stable and level.

4. Fully extend the knee of the leg on the pedal throughout the exercise since the objective is on the two-joint gastrocnemius, not the soleus or other one-joint plantar flexors.

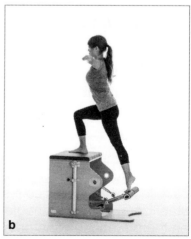

b

FULL PIKE

Primary Muscles Involved

Abdominals and serratus anterior

Objectives

Abdominal strength, scapular stabilization, and shoulder girdle strength and control

Indications

This is a very challenging exercise that gets deep into the abdominals. The combination of shoulder girdle muscle activation and stabilization with such deep core work often allows people to really feel the abdominals working more intensely than ever before. The strength, control, muscle integration, and focus required to do this correctly is similar to that of a handstand.

Precautions or Contraindications

Acute shoulder injury or pain, acute back injury or pain, lumbar disk pathology, or osteoporosis

Resistance

Medium (another exercise in which less resistance is more difficult)

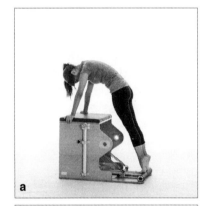

Instructions

Stand on the pedal facing the chair, with the hands placed at the far edge of the seat, fingers facing out. Align the shoulders directly over the wrists. Draw the scapulae down and back, pressing down into the chair to activate the serratus anterior. Engage the deepest abdominals to pull into a *C*-curve position (see photo *a*). Exhale to draw the abdominals up and in even deeper, raising the pedal to the very top (see photos *b* and *c*). Inhale to lower the pedal almost to the floor, keeping the pike position.

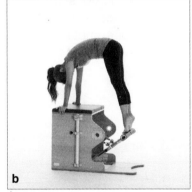

Variations

1. Even if a client is unable to do the full pike, floating up a few inches (several cm) from the pike position to get the coordination and feeling of deep abdominal activation is very valuable.

2. Perform a side pike, which targets the oblique abdominal muscles. Stand on the

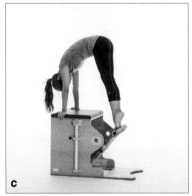

pedal sideways with the inside leg in front and the hands holding the edge of the chair (see photos *d* and *e*). Follow the instructions for full pike.

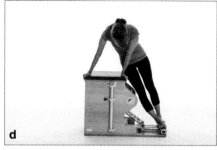

Progression

Perform a single-leg pike by holding one leg out to the side in hip abduction. This can be done in either full pike or side pike versions.

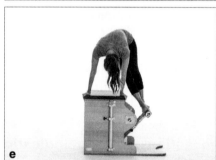

Technique Tips

1. Use the deepest core muscles to pull up into maximum lumbar flexion. Pull the pelvis toward the head and the head toward the pelvis, as if trying to make the shape of the body as small as possible.
2. Keep the shoulders over the hands and the head aligned with the spine. Do not let the shoulders shift forward to lift the body.
3. Imagine the body floating up with the pedals, as if levitating.
4. If it is impossible to float the body, add resistance to assist so the patient can experience the movement and feeling. The inability to do this exercise is often not an issue of strength but of neuromuscular integration.

PILATES FOR COMMON INJURIES AND PATHOLOGIES

The Cervical and Thoracic Spine

Neck pain is very common and has many causes: stress or tension, prolonged postures, minor falls or accidents, referred pain from upper back injuries, overuse (muscular strain), and simply aging. In fact, two thirds of all adults experience neck pain at some point in their lifetime (Cote et al. 2008), and neck pain is the second most common disorder relating to injury and disability claims (Childs et. al 2004).

Pilates is ideal for neck injuries and cervical pathologies because of the emphasis on good posture, proper breathing, and muscle elongation. In working with the cervical spine, we must also consider the upper thoracic region, clavicle, and scapula—due the muscular and facial relationships. In general, most exercises that target scapular and shoulder stabilization and mobility will also be appropriate for cervical pathologies. See the following tables for information on how to apply this to specific conditions.

Note that these tables represent what would be generally appropriate for patients with the associated diagnoses or pathologies. However, as every person will present differently and have different issues, it is crucial to assess each client individually and either omit exercises or choose the correct modification as appropriate. If the client does not have the strength, flexibility, or control to perform an exercise correctly, it should not be included in his program.

Exercise Recommendations for Common Cervical Injuries and Pathologies

CERVICAL DISK PATHOLOGIES			
Pathology	General contraindications and precautions	Common problems	Goals
Disk • Degeneration • Protrusion • Herniation	• Avoid deep flexion, compression (vertical loading), and severe rotation.	• Neck pain • Upper spinal instability • Upper core weakness • Tight upper trapezius, levator scapulae • Poor posture (forward head, rounded shoulder) • Peripheral symptoms (arm pain, numbness, tingling, or weakness)	• Retrain upper quadrant • Strengthen upper core with the cervical spine in neutral • Improve cervical and scapular stabilization • Improve flexibility of tight neck or shoulder muscles • Improve posture • Increase core strength

Recommended exercises

MAT

Single-leg lifts, Supine spine twist, Pre-hundred prep, Modified single-leg stretch, Front support, Leg pull front, Side bend, Basic back extension, Sphinx, Goalpost, Swimming

REFORMER

Footwork (headrest down), Arms supine series, Single-arm coordination, Ab openings (head down variation), Hip work series, Seated Biceps, Rhomboids 1, Rhomboids 2, Goalpost rotator cuff, Bilateral external rotation, Chest expansion wide, Hug a tree, Modified rows, Chest expansion, Shoulder internal rotation, Shoulder external rotation, Shoulder diagonal pull, Arms overhead, Arm circles, Kneeling biceps, Quadruped abs, Reverse quadruped abs, Quadruped triceps kickback, Up stretch 1, Up stretch 2, Long stretch, Up stretch 3, Down stretch, Shoulder push, Prone pulling straps 1, Prone pulling straps 2

CADILLAC

Hip work: double leg supine series, Supine hip flexor stretch with manual assist, Supine protraction and retraction on foam roll, Single-leg side series, Seated protraction and retraction, Push-through sitting stretches, Standing arm work series

WUNDA CHAIR

Modified swan on floor, Single-arm push-up, Reverse shrugs, Triceps press sit, Prone triceps, Basic swan, Torso press sit, Full pike

CERVICAL OR THORACIC OSTEOARTHRITIS			
Pathology	**General contraindications and precautions**	**Common problems**	**Goals**
Osteoarthritis • Osteoarthrosis • Degenerative joint disease • Spondylosis	• Avoid high-impact exercises. • Go easy (less resistance) during periods of inflammation or pain.	• Neck pain • Neck stiffness • Limited range of motion • Symptoms worse in the morning • Upper spinal instability • Upper core weakness • Tight upper trapezius, levator scapulae, superficial anterior neck muscles • Poor posture (forward head, rounded shoulders)	• Retrain upper quadrant • Improve cervical and scapular stabilization • Improve flexibility of tight neck or shoulder muscles • Improve posture • Increase core strength

Recommended exercises

MAT

Pelvic curl, Single-leg lifts, Supine spine twist, Chest lift (variation 2), Chest lift with rotation (variation 2), Pre-hundred prep, Modified single-leg stretch, Front support, Leg pull front, Side bend, Basic back extension (prep variation), Sphinx, Goalpost, Swimming

REFORMER

Footwork, Bottom lift, Bottom lift with extension, Arms supine series, Single-arm coordination, Ab openings (head down variation), Hip work series, Seated Biceps, Rhomboids 1, Rhomboids 2, Goalpost rotator cuff, Bilateral external rotation, Chest expansion wide, Hug a tree, Modified rows, Chest expansion, Shoulder internal rotation, Shoulder external rotation, Shoulder diagonal pull, Arms overhead, Arm circles, Kneeling biceps, Quadruped abs, Reverse quadruped abs, Quadruped triceps kickback, Up stretch 1, Up stretch 2, Long stretch, Up stretch 3, Down stretch, Shoulder push, Modified balance control front, Prone pulling straps 1, Prone pulling straps 2, Quadratus lumborum stretch

CADILLAC

Pelvic curl with roll-up bar (RUB), Breathing with push-through bar (PTB), Hip work: double leg supine series, Supine hip flexor stretch with manual assist, Supine protraction and retraction on foam roll, Single leg side series, Seated protraction and retraction, Push-through sitting stretches, Standing arm work series

WUNDA CHAIR

Pelvic curl, Modified swan on floor, Single-arm push-up, Reverse shrugs, Triceps press sit, Prone triceps, Basic swan, Torso press sit, Full pike

CERVICAL STENOSIS			
Pathology	**General contraindications and precautions**	**Common problems**	**Goals**
Stenosis	• Use caution with cervical extension. • Avoid cervical extension if it brings on pain, numbness, or tingling.	• Long history of pain in the neck, shoulder blade, arm, or hand • Poor posture • Numbness, tingling, or weakness in one or both arms • Neck stiffness • Limited range of motion • Upper spinal instability • Upper core weakness • Tight upper trapezius or levator scapulae	• Work in flexion first, but progress to neutral positions and mild extension when the patient is symptom free • Retrain upper quadrant • Increase cervical and scapular stabilization • Improve flexibility of tight neck and shoulder muscles • Improve posture • Increase core strength

Recommended exercises

MAT

Pelvic curl, Single-leg lifts, Supine spine twist, Chest lift (variation 2), Chest lift with rotation (variation 2), Pre-hundred prep, Modified single-leg stretch, Front support, Leg pull front, Side bend, Sphinx, Goalpost

REFORMER

Footwork (headrest up and holding dowel with palms up), Bottom lift, Bottom lift with extension, Arms supine series, Single-arm coordination, Ab openings (head down variation), Hip work series, Seated Biceps, Rhomboids 1, Rhomboids 2, Goalpost rotator cuff, Bilateral external rotation, Chest expansion wide, Hug a tree, Modified rows, Chest expansion, Shoulder internal rotation, Shoulder external rotation, Shoulder diagonal pull, Arms overhead, Arm circles, Kneeling biceps, Quadruped abs, Reverse quadruped abs, Quadruped triceps kickback, Up stretch 1, Up stretch 2, Long stretch, Up stretch 3, Shoulder push, Modified balance control front

CADILLAC

Pelvic curl with RUB, Breathing with PTB, Hip work: double leg supine series, Supine hip flexor stretch with manual assist, Supine protraction and retraction on foam roll, Single-leg side series, Seated protraction and retraction, Push-through sitting stretches, Standing arm work series

WUNDA CHAIR

Pelvic curl, Single-arm push-up, Reverse shrugs, Triceps press sit, Prone triceps, Full pike

THORACIC OUTLET SYNDROME			
Pathology	General contraindications and precautions	Common problems	Goals
Thoracic outlet syndrome	• Aggravated by compression of the thoracic outlet region. • Avoid any positions or movements that reproduce symptoms in the patient's arm.	• Numbness, tingling, pain • Ablation of the radial pulse • Coldness in the affected arm • Poor posture • Tight or dysfunctional scalene muscles • Lack of sufficient cervical or scapular stabilization	• Decrease compression at thoracic outlet • Increase flexibility and restore normal function of scalene muscles • Retrain upper quadrant • Improve cervical and scapular stabilization • Improve flexibility of tight neck and shoulder muscles • Improve posture • Increase core strength

Recommended exercises

MAT

Pelvic curl, Single-leg lifts, Supine spine twist, Chest lift (variation 2 or 4), Chest lift with rotation (variation 2 or 4), Pre-hundred prep, Modified single-leg stretch, Front support (on elbows), Leg pull front (on elbows), Side bend (on elbow), Basic back extension, Sphinx, Goalpost

REFORMER

Footwork (pad shoulder rests and hold dowel with palms up), Arms supine series, Single-arm coordination, Ab openings (head down variation), Hip work series, Rhomboids 1, Rhomboids 2, Goalpost rotator cuff, Bilateral external rotation, Chest expansion wide, Modified rows, Chest expansion, Shoulder internal rotation, Shoulder external rotation, Kneeling biceps, Quadruped abs, Reverse quadruped abs, Quadruped triceps kickback, Up stretch 2, Long stretch, Up stretch 3, Down stretch, Shoulder push, Modified balance control front, Prone pulling straps 1, Prone pulling straps 2

CADILLAC

Pelvic curl with RUB, Breathing with PTB, Hip work: double leg supine series, Supine hip flexor stretch with manual assist, Supine protraction and retraction on foam roll, Single-leg side series, Seated protraction and retraction, Push-through sitting stretches, from the Standing arm work series: Chest expansion, Biceps

WUNDA CHAIR

Pelvic curl, Reverse shrugs, Triceps press sit, Prone triceps, Basic swan, Torso press sit

WHIPLASH INJURY			
Pathology	**General contraindications and precautions**	**Common problems**	**Goals**
Whiplash injury	• Avoid positions or movements that cause tension in the neck muscles.	• Neck and upper back pain • Headaches • Inhibited upper quadrant • Upper spinal instability • Tight upper trapezius, levator scapulae, sternocleidomastoid, scalene muscles • Poor posture (forward head, rounded shoulders) • Sensory disturbances in arms	• Retrain upper quadrant • Improve cervical and scapular stabilization • Improve flexibility of tight neck and shoulder muscles • Improve posture • Increase core strength

Recommended exercises

MAT

Single-leg lifts, Supine spine twist, Pre-hundred prep, Modified single-leg stretch, Front support (on elbows), Leg pull front (on elbows), Side bend (on elbow), Basic back extension (prep variation), Sphinx, Goalpost

REFORMER

Footwork (hold dowel with palms up), Arms supine series, Single-arm coordination, Ab openings (head down variation), Hip work series, Bilateral external rotation, Chest expansion wide, Hug a tree, Modified rows, Chest expansion, Shoulder internal rotation, Shoulder external rotation, Kneeling biceps, Quadruped abs, Reverse quadruped abs, Quadruped triceps kickback, Up stretch 1, Up stretch 2, Shoulder push, Quadratus lumborum stretch

CADILLAC

Hip work: double leg supine series, Supine hip flexor stretch with manual assist, Supine protraction and retraction on foam roll, Single-leg side series, Seated protraction and retraction, Push-through sitting stretches, From the Standing arm work series: Chest expansion, Hug a tree, Biceps

WUNDA CHAIR

Pelvic curl, Single-arm push-up (quadruped position only), Reverse shrugs, Triceps press sit, Prone triceps, Basic swan, Piriformis stretch

OSTEOPOROSIS			
Pathology	**General contraindications and precautions**	**Common problems**	**Goals**
Osteoporosis	• Avoid spinal flexion. • Avoid all forms of rollups and crunches. • Avoid abdominal work with oblique rotation. • Avoid pressure on the rib cage. • Avoid weight bearing on the cervical or thoracic spine. • Limit spinal rotation and lateral flexion. • Avoid forced external rotation of the hip.	• Reduction in bone mineral density of >25% leads to four to eight times greater risk of fracture • Poor posture • Thoracic kyphosis • Height loss	• Increase bone mineral density with weight-bearing exercises • Focus on thoracic extension to improve posture and reduce the risk of fractures • Retrain upper quadrant • Improve cervical and scapular stabilization • Improve flexibility of tight neck and shoulder muscles • Improve balance and proprioception (to reduce risk of falls that lead to fractures) • Increase core strength

Recommended exercises

MAT

Pelvic curl, Single-leg lifts, Supine spine twist (variations 1 and 2), Chest lift (variation 3 only) Pre-hundred prep, Modified single-leg stretch, Front support, Leg pull front, Side bend, Basic back extension, Sphinx, Goalpost, Swimming

REFORMER

Footwork (with heavy spring and holding dowel with palms up), Arms supine series, Single-arm coordination, Ab openings (head down variation), Hip work series, Seated biceps, Rhomboids 1, Rhomboids 2, Goalpost rotator cuff, Bilateral external rotation, Chest expansion wide, Hug a tree, Modified rows, Chest expansion, Shoulder internal rotation, Should external rotation, Shoulder diagonal pull, Arms overhead, Arm circles, Kneeling biceps, Quadruped abs (flat back only), Reverse quadruped abs (flat back only), Quadruped triceps kickback, Up stretch 1, Up stretch 2, Long stretch, Up stretch 3, Down stretch, Shoulder push, Modified balance control front, Skating hybrid, Side splits, Terminal knee extension (standing), Hamstring curl (standing), Scooter (flat back variation only), Standing lunge, Prone pulling straps 1, Prone pulling straps 2

CADILLAC

Pelvic curl with RUB, Hip work: double leg supine series, Supine hip flexor stretch with manual assist, Supine protraction and retraction on foam roll, Single-leg side series, Seated protraction and retraction, Assisted squats, Resisted lunges, Standing arm work series

WUNDA CHAIR

Modified swan on floor, Single-arm push-up, Reverse shrugs, Triceps press sit, Prone triceps, Basic swan, Torso press sit, Calf press, Standing leg press, Forward lunge, Backward step-down, Calf press in forward lunge

10

The Lumbar Spine

Low back pain is a very common, disabling, and costly health problem. One quarter of all physical therapy visits in the United States involve patients with low back pain. It has been estimated that 80 percent of adults at least once in their lives will suffer an episode of back pain severe enough to make them stop working temporarily (Limba da Fonseca, Magini, and de Freitas 2009). Machado et. al (2017) report that one-third of patients will experience recurrent low back pain, whereas other researchers have reported recurrence rates as high as 60-80% (Troup, Martin, and Lloyd. 1981). There is no evidence to support that modalities commonly used in rehabilitation such as medication, ultrasound, laser, heat and ice, traction, or electrical stimulation really affect the long-term outcomes of low back pain. Exercise, however, has been shown to reduce pain and disability in people suffering from low back pain. Please refer to chapter 1 for research studies advocating the use of the Pilates method as the exercise of choice for patients with low back pain. Depending on the cause of the low back pain, the specific exercise prescription will vary. See the following tables for exercise prescriptions for low back pain and the lumbar spine.

Note that these tables represent what would be generally appropriate for patients with the associated diagnoses and pathologies. However, as every person will present differently and have different issues, it is crucial to assess each client individually and either omit exercises or choose the correct modification as appropriate. If the client does not have the strength, flexibility, or control to perform an exercise correctly, it should not be included in his program.

Exercise Recommendations for Common Lumbar Injuries and Pathologies

LUMBAR DISK PATHOLOGIES			
Pathology	**General contraindications and precautions**	**Common problems**	**Goals**
Disk • Degeneration • Protrusion • Herniation	• Avoid deep lumbar flexion. • Avoid compression (vertical loading). • Avoid severe rotation.	• Low back pain • Spinal instability • Core weakness • Hamstring or hip flexor tightness • Poor posture • Peripheral symptoms (leg pain, numbness, tingling)	• Unload disk • Extension-based exercises • Core stabilization • Increase strength • Improve lower extremity (LE) flexibility • Improve posture

Recommended exercises

MAT

Pelvic curl (neutral position variation only), Single-leg lifts, Supine spine twist, Chest lift (variation 3 only), Chest lift with rotation (variation 3 only), Pre-hundred prep, Modified single-leg stretch, Front support, Leg pull front, Side bend (variation 1), Basic back extension, Sphinx, Goalpost, Shoulder bridge prep, Shoulder bridge

REFORMER

Footwork, Bottom lift (variation 1 only), Bottom lift with extension (neutral spine variation only), Arms supine series, Single-arm coordination, Ab openings (head down variation), Hip work series, Adductor stretch, Hamstring stretch, Quadruped abs (flat back variation only), Reverse quadruped abs (flat back variation only), Scooter (flat back variation only), Standing lunge, Seated biceps (kneeling position preferred), Rhomboids 1 (kneeling position preferred), Rhomboids 2 (kneeling position preferred), Bilateral external rotation (kneeling position preferred), Chest expansion wide (kneeling position preferred), Hug a tree (kneeling position preferred), Quadruped triceps kickback, Modified rows, Chest expansion, Shoulder diagonal pull, Arm circles, Kneeling biceps, Prone pulling straps 1, Prone pulling straps 2, Long stretch, Down stretch, Modified balance control front, Side splits, Skating hybrid, Jumping series, Quadratus lumborum stretch

CADILLAC

Breathing with (PTB) (neutral position variation), Hip work: double leg supine series, Supine hip flexor stretch with manual assist, Single-leg side series, Assisted squats, Resisted lunges, Standing arm work series

WUNDA CHAIR

Hamstring curl, Modified swan on floor, Single-arm push-up, Prone triceps, Basic swan, Calf press, Standing leg press, Forward lunge, Backward step-down, Calf press in forward lunge

LUMBOSACRAL OSTEOARTHRITIS			
Pathology	General contraindications and precautions	Common problems	Goals
Osteoarthritis • Osteoarthrosis • Degenerative joint disease • Spondylosis	• Avoid high-impact exercises. • Reduce intensity when symptomatic.	• Pain • Stiffness • Restricted range of motion • Core weakness • Poor posture	• Improve spinal articulation and mobility • Improve flexibility • Core stabilization • Increase strength • Improve posture

Recommended exercises

MAT

Pelvic curl, Single-leg lifts, Supine spine twist, Chest lift, Chest lift with rotation, Hundred prep, Pre-hundred prep, Single-leg stretch, Modified single-leg stretch, Front support, Leg pull front, Side bend, Basic back extension, Sphinx, Goalpost, Shoulder bridge prep, Shoulder bridge

REFORMER

Footwork, Bottom lift, Bottom lift with extension, Arms supine series, Hundred prep, Hundred, Coordination, Single-arm coordination, Ab openings, Hip work series, Adductor stretch, Hamstring stretch, Quadruped abs, Reverse quadruped abs, Scooter, Standing lunge, Quadratus lumborum stretch, Seated biceps, Rhomboids 1, Rhomboids 2, Bilateral external rotation, Chest expansion wide, Hug a tree, Quadruped triceps kickback, Modified rows, Chest expansion (begin with long box variation), Shoulder diagonal pull, Arm circles (begin with long box variation), Kneeling biceps (begin with long box variation), Prone pulling straps 1, Prone pulling straps 2, Up stretch 1, Up stretch 2, Up stretch 3, Down stretch, Skating hybrid, Side splits, Quadratus lumborum stretch

CADILLAC

Pelvic curl with RUB, Breathing with PTB, Hip work: double leg supine series, Supine hip flexor stretch with manual assist, Supine protraction and retraction on foam roll, Single-leg side series, Push-through sitting stretches, Assisted squats, Resisted lunges, Standing arm work series

WUNDA CHAIR

Pelvic curl, Hamstring curl, Modified swan on floor, Reverse shrugs, Triceps press sit, Prone triceps, Basic swan, Piriformis stretch, Standing leg press

LUMBAR STENOSIS			
Pathology	**General contraindications and precautions**	**Common problems**	**Goals**
Stenosis	• Use caution with lumbar extension. • Avoid lumbar extension if it brings on pain, numbness, or tingling.	• Long history of pain in back, buttocks, or legs • Heaviness, weakness in buttocks or legs • Numbness or tingling down legs • Pain increased by walking or standing upright • Stiffness • Restricted range of motion • Antalgic gait	• Work in flexion first, but progress to neutral and mild extension when symptom free • Improve LE flexibility • Core stabilization • Increase strength • Improve posture

Recommended exercises

MAT

Pelvic curl, Single-leg lifts, Supine spine twist, Chest lift (variation 1), Chest lift with rotation (variation 1), Hundred prep, Pre-hundred prep, Modified single-leg stretch, Front support, Side bend, Sphinx (variation over physio ball), Shoulder bridge prep

REFORMER

Footwork, Bottom lift, Arms supine series (start with series variation 1), Hundred prep, Coordination, Ab openings, Hip work series, Adductor stretch, Hamstring stretch, Quadruped abs (round back variation), Reverse quadruped abs, Scooter, Quadratus lumborum stretch, Seated biceps, Rhomboids 1, Rhomboids 2, Bilateral external rotation, Chest expansion wide, Hug a tree, Quadruped triceps kickback, Modified rows, Chest expansion (begin with long box variation), Shoulder diagonal pull, Arm circles (begin with long box variation), Kneeling biceps (begin with long box variation), Up stretch 1, Up stretch 2, Shoulder push, Skating hybrid

CADILLAC

Pelvic curl with RUB, Breathing with PTB, Hip work: double leg supine, Supine hip flexor stretch with manual assist, Supine protraction and retraction on foam roll, Push-through sitting stretches (part 1 only), Assisted squats

WUNDA CHAIR

Pelvic curl, Hamstring curl, Single-arm push-up, Reverse shrugs, Triceps press sit, Piriformis stretch, Standing leg press, Full pike (variation 1)

SPONDYLOLISTHESIS			
Pathology	**General contraindications and precautions**	**Common problems**	**Goals**
Spondylolisthesis	• Avoid extension. • Use caution with extreme positions or ranges of motion.	• Spinal instability • Pain • Stiffness • Intermittent shocks of pain down leg(s) • Tight hamstrings • Forward lean during gait • Core weakness • Poor posture	• Lumbo-pelvic stabilization • Increase core strength • Always work in flexion or neutral • Improve posture • Increase strength

Recommended exercises

MAT

Pelvic curl, Single-leg lifts, Supine spine twist, Chest lift (variation 1), Chest lift with rotation (variation 1), Hundred prep, Hundred (variations only), Pre-hundred prep, Single-leg stretch, Front support, Side bend, Sphinx (variation over physio ball *only*), Shoulder bridge prep

REFORMER

Footwork, Bottom lift, Arms supine series (series variation 1), Hundred prep, Coordination, Hip work series, Adductor stretch, Hamstring stretch, Quadruped abs (round back *only*), Reverse quadruped abs (round back *only*), Scooter (round back *only*), Seated biceps, Rhomboids 1, Rhomboids 2, Bilateral external rotation, Chest expansion wide, Hug a tree, Quadruped triceps kickback, Modified rows (long box variation), Chest expansion (long box variation), Shoulder diagonal pull, Arm circles (long box variation), Kneeling biceps (long box variation), Up stretch 1, Up stretch 2, Shoulder push, Skating hybrid

CADILLAC

Pelvic curl with RUB, Breathing with PTB, Hip work: double leg supine series, Supine hip flexor stretch with manual assist, Supine protraction and retraction on foam roll, Push through sitting stretches (part 1 only), Assisted squats

WUNDA CHAIR

Pelvic curl, Hamstring curl, Single-arm push-up (quadruped position only), Reverse shrugs, Triceps press sit, Piriformis stretch, Standing leg press, Backward step-down

LUMBOSACRAL FACET JOINT SYNDROME			
Pathology	**General contraindications and precautions**	**Common problems**	**Goals**
Lumbosacral facet joint syndrome	• Avoid positions of pain.	• Low back pain (localized, worse in certain positions based on location of lesion) • Restricted range of motion • Poor posture • Stiffness • Muscle tightness (long back extensors)	• Restore normal range of motion • Improve LE flexibility • Improve core stabilization • Increase strength • Improve posture • Improve spinal articulation and mobility

Recommended exercises

MAT

Pelvic curl, Single leg lifts, Supine spine twist, Chest lift (start with variation 1), Chest lift with rotation (start with variation 1), Hundred prep, Hundred, Pre-hundred prep, Single-leg stretch, Modified single-leg stretch, Front support, Leg pull front, Side bend (caution: may be painful depending on site of lesion), Basic back extension, Swimming, Sphinx, Goalpost, Shoulder bridge prep, Shoulder bridge

REFORMER

Footwork, Bottom lift, Bottom lift with extension, Arms supine series, Hundred prep, Hundred, Coordination, Single-arm coordination, Ab openings, Hip work series, Adductor stretch, Hamstring stretch, Scooter, Standing lunge, Quadratus lumborum stretch, Seated biceps, Rhomboids 1, Rhomboids 2, Bilateral external rotation, Chest expansion wide, Hug a tree, Quadruped triceps kickback, Modified rows, Chest expansion, Shoulder diagonal pull, Arm circles, Kneeling biceps, Prone pulling straps 1, Prone pulling straps 2, Up stretch 1, Up stretch 2, Up stretch 3, Long stretch, Down stretch, Shoulder push, Skating hybrid, Side splits, Jumping series

CADILLAC

Pelvic curl with RUB, Breathing with PTB, Hip work: double leg supine series, Supine hip flexor stretch with manual assist, Supine protraction and retraction on foam roll, Single-leg side series, Push-through sitting stretches, Assisted squats, Standing arm work series

WUNDA CHAIR

Pelvic curl, Hamstring curl, Modified swan on floor, Single-arm push-up, Reverse shrugs, Triceps press sit, Prone triceps, Basic swan, Torso press sit, Piriformis stretch, Standing leg press

POSTURAL SYNDROME			
Pathology	**General contraindications and precautions**	**Common problems**	**Goals**
Postural syndrome	None	• Low back pain • Poor posture • Core weakness • Lumbosacral instability • Tight hip flexors • Tight hamstrings • Stiffness	• Improve posture • Improve LE flexibility • Core stabilization • Increase strength • Improve spinal articulation and mobility
Recommended exercises			
All			

SCIATICA			
Pathology	**General contraindications and precautions**	**Common problems**	**Goals**
Sciatica • Compression of the sciatic nerve caused by disk herniation, stenosis, or bone spurs	• Specific contraindications and precautions depend on the source of nerve compression. Most often, disk pathology is the cause, so follow disk precautions. • Avoid deep lumbar flexion, compression (vertical loading), and severe rotation.	• Pain in the low back that radiates down from buttocks to the back of one thigh and leg to the foot • Spinal instability • Core weakness • Hamstring and hip flexor tightness • Poor posture • Other peripheral symptoms (numbness, tingling down the leg)	• Unload disk • Core stabilization • Increase strength • Improve LE flexibility • Improve posture

Recommended exercises

MAT

Pelvic curl (neutral position variation only), Single-leg lifts, Supine spine twist, Chest lift (variation 3 only), Chest lift with rotation (variation 3 only), Pre-hundred prep, Modified single-leg stretch, Front support, Leg pull front, Side bend (variation 1), Basic back extension, Swimming, Sphinx, Goalpost, Shoulder bridge prep, Shoulder bridge

REFORMER

Footwork, Bottom lift (variation 1 only), Bottom lift with extension (neutral spine variation only), Arms supine series, Single-arm coordination, Ab openings (head down variation), Hip work series, Adductor stretch, Hamstring stretch, Quadruped abs (flat back variation only), Reverse quadruped abs (flat back variation only), Scooter (flat back variation only), Standing lunge, Seated biceps, Rhomboids 1, Rhomboids 2, Bilateral external rotation, Chest expansion wide, Hug a tree, Quadruped triceps kickback, Modified rows, Chest expansion, Shoulder diagonal pull, Arm circles, Kneeling biceps, Prone pulling straps 1, Prone pulling straps 2, Long stretch, Down stretch, Side splits, Skating hybrid, Jumping series

CADILLAC

Breathing with PTB (neutral position variation), Hip work: double leg supine series, Supine hip flexor stretch with manual assist, Single-leg side series, Assisted squats, Resisted lunges, Standing arm work series

WUNDA CHAIR

Hamstring curl, Modified swan on floor, Single-arm push-up, Prone triceps, Basic swan, Standing leg press, Forward lunge, Backward step-down

SACROILIAC JOINT DYSFUNCTION			
Pathology	**General contraindications and precautions**	**Common problems**	**Goals**
Sacroiliac joint dysfunction • Instability or hypomobility	• Avoid unilateral weight-bearing exercises when symptomatic. • Avoid bottom-lift or bridging exercises in the acute stage.	• Pain in low back and buttock area and often referred to groin or posterior thigh • Pain aggravated by unilateral weight bearing (standing on one leg, walking, stairs) • Lumbosacral instability • Tight hamstrings, hip flexors, or piriformis • Weak gluteal muscles	• Improve lumbopelvic stabilization • Increase core strength • Strengthen gluteal muscles • Improve posture • Improve LE flexibility

Recommended exercises

MAT

Single-leg lifts, Supine spine twist, Chest lift, Chest lift with rotation, Hundred prep, Hundred, Pre-hundred prep, Single leg stretch, Modified single-leg stretch, Front support, Leg pull front, Side bend, Basic back extension, Swimming

REFORMER

Footwork, Arms supine series, Hundred prep, Hundred, Coordination, Single-arm coordination, Ab openings, Hip work series, Adductor stretch, Hamstring stretch, Quadruped abs, Reverse quadruped abs, Quadratus lumborum stretch, Seated biceps, Rhomboids 1, Rhomboids 2, Bilateral external rotation, Chest expansion wide, Hug a tree, Quadruped triceps kickback, Modified rows, Chest expansion, Shoulder diagonal pull, Arm circles, Kneeling biceps, Prone pulling straps 1, Prone pulling straps 2, Up stretch 1, Up stretch 2, Up stretch 3, Long stretch, Down stretch, Shoulder push, Skating hybrid[a]

CADILLAC

Hip work: double leg supine series, Supine hip flexor stretch with manual assist, Single-leg side series, Push-through sitting stretches, Assisted squats, Resisted Lunges[a], Standing arm work series

WUNDA CHAIR

Hamstring curl, Modified swan on floor, Single-arm push-up, Reverse shrugs, Triceps press sit, Prone triceps, Basic swan, Piriformis stretch, Standing leg press[a], Full Lunge[a], Backward step-down[a], Full pike

[a] Not appropriate for acute cases

11

The Shoulder

When referring to the shoulder complex we are not just talking about the glenohumeral joint. We must consider the entire region: three bones (humerus, clavicle, and scapula), four joints (glenohumeral, acromioclavicular, sternoclavicular, and scapulothoracic), and numerous muscles. The glenohumeral joint is the most mobile joint in the human body. With the complexity of this region and the extreme mobility comes a lack of stability and thus a high risk of injury. All of the muscles of the shoulder girdle must work together to provide a coordination of movement called scapulohumeral rhythm. This involves stabilization of the scapula, elevation of the humerus by the deltoid, and the deltoid counterforce provided by the rotator cuff to keep the humeral head depressed in the glenohumeral joint so that impingement does not occur. When all of these movements happen appropriately, the shoulder can be elevated overhead without pain.

Without correct mechanics it is likely that at some point problems will occur in the shoulder, or in related areas such as the neck or back. This may take the form of tendinopathy, muscle tear, dislocation, or simply overuse of other muscle groups such as the upper trapezius, which in turn can lead to neck and shoulder tension. As reviewed in chapter 1, several studies have found that poor thoracic posture, abnormal shoulder biomechanics, and scapular instability are often a cause or effect of neck–shoulder disorders. The results of the study done by Emery et al. (2010) provided evidence to support that Pilates training could help prevent such disorders.

Many Pilates exercises, especially in the advanced repertoire, place great demands on the shoulder joint. Therefore, a clear understanding of shoulder mechanics is essential to be able to teach these exercises correctly and avoid injury. At the same time, with many Pilates exercises being closed chain, and some even unilateral closed chain, Pilates, when used correctly, is an excellent way to achieve scapular stabilization and thus strong, healthy shoulders; see the following tables.

Note that these tables represent what would be generally appropriate for patients with the associated diagnoses or pathologies. However, as every person will present differently and have different issues, it is crucial to assess each client individually and either omit exercises or choose the correct modification as appropriate. If the client does not have the strength, flexibility, or control to perform an exercise correctly, it should not be included in her program.

Exercise Recommendations for Common Shoulder Injuries and Pathologies

IMPINGEMENT SYNDROME, BURSITIS, AND TENDINITIS			
Pathology	General contraindications and precautions	Common problems	Goals
Impingement syndrome Bursitis Tendinitis	• Avoid overhead reaching or lifting.	• Pain when reaching the arm overhead • Pain when reaching the arm backwards • Poor posture (forward head, rounded shoulder) • Poor scapular stabilization • Shoulder hypermobility • Poor biomechanics (dysfunctional scapulohumeral rhythm)	• Increase strength of scapular stabilizers • Strengthen rotator cuff muscles • Improve posture (strengthen muscles that draw shoulders down and back) • Stretch muscles that pull the shoulders forward • Restore normal scapulohumeral rhythm • Increase core strength

Recommended exercises

MAT

Pelvic curl, Single-leg lifts, Supine spine twist, Chest lift (variation 4), Chest lift with rotation (variation 4), Hundred prep, Hundred, Single-leg stretch, Front support (on elbows), Leg pull front (on elbows), Side bend (on elbow), Basic back extension, Sphinx, Shoulder bridge prep, Shoulder bridge

REFORMER

Footwork, Bottom lift, Bottom lift with extension, Arms supine series, Hundred prep, Hundred, Coordination, Single-arm coordination, Ab openings, Hip work series, Quadruped abs, Reverse quadruped abs, Scooter, Seated biceps, Rhomboids 1, Rhomboids 2, Bilateral external rotation, Chest expansion wide, Hug a tree, Quadruped triceps kickback, Modified rows, Chest expansion, Shoulder internal rotation, Shoulder external rotation, Kneeling biceps, Prone pulling straps 1, Prone pulling straps 2, Down stretch, Shoulder push, Modified balance control front

CADILLAC

Pelvic curl with RUB, Supine protraction and retraction on foam roll, Assisted squats, Standing arm work series, Chest expansion, Hug a tree, Biceps

WUNDA CHAIR

Pelvic curl, Single-arm push-up, Reverse shrugs, Triceps press sit, Prone triceps, Basic swan, Torso press sit, Full pike

ROTATOR CUFF INJURY			
Pathology	**General contraindications and precautions**	**Common problems**	**Goals**
Rotator cuff injury • Rotator cuff tear • Status post–rotator cuff repair • For post-op rotator cuff repair, follow specific physician protocol for when to begin exercises	• Avoid overhead reaching or lifting.	• Shoulder pain worse with elevating arm overhead or reaching backward • Night pain • Pain radiating into lateral arm • Weakness of shoulder and arm muscles • Forward head or rounded shoulder posture • Poor scapular stabilization • Poor scapulohumeral rhythm	• Increase strength of scapular stabilizers • Improve posture (strengthen muscles that draw the shoulders down and back) • Stretch muscles that pull the shoulders forward • Strengthen rotator cuff • Restore full range of motion • Restore normal scapulohumeral rhythm • Increase core strength

Recommended exercises

MAT

Pelvic curl, Single-leg lifts, Supine spine twist, Chest lift (variation 4), Chest lift with rotation (variation 4), Hundred prep, Hundred, Pre-hundred prep, Single-leg stretch, Front support (on elbows), Leg pull front (on elbows), Side bend (on elbow), Basic back extension, Sphinx, Goalpost, Shoulder bridge prep, Shoulder bridge

REFORMER

Footwork (hold dowel with palms up), Bottom lift, Bottom lift with extension, Arms supine series, Hundred prep, Hundred, Coordination, Single-arm coordination, Ab openings, Hip work series, Quadruped abs, Reverse quadruped abs, Scooter, Seated biceps, Bilateral external rotation, Chest expansion wide, Quadruped triceps kickback, Modified rows, Chest expansion, Shoulder internal rotation, Shoulder external rotation, Kneeling biceps, Prone pulling straps 1, Prone pulling straps 2, Down stretch, Shoulder push, Modified balance control front

CADILLAC

Pelvic curl with RUB, Supine protraction and retraction on foam roll, Seated protraction and retraction, Assisted squats, Standing arm work series: Chest expansion, Hug a tree, Biceps

WUNDA CHAIR

Pelvic curl, Single-arm push-up (quadruped position), Reverse shrugs, Triceps press sit, Prone triceps, Basic swan

FROZEN SHOULDER			
Pathology	**General contraindications and precautions**	**Common problems**	**Goals**
Adhesive capsulitis (frozen shoulder)	• Avoid exercises that cause any pain. • Do not force any range of motion.	• Extremely limited range of motion (especially in external rotation and abduction • Shoulder and arm pain, worsened with movement • Shoulder joint stiffness • Scapular hypomobility • Rounded shoulder and often forward head posture • Shoulder muscle atrophy or weakness • Difficulty or inability with activities of daily living (such as brushing hair or hooking bra)	• Scapular mobilization • Strengthen shoulder musculature in pain-free positions • Improve posture • Restore normal range of motion and scapulohumeral rhythm • Increase core strength

Recommended exercises

MAT

Pelvic curl, Single-leg lifts, Supine spine twist, Chest lift (variation 4), Chest lift with rotation (variation 4), Hundred prep, Hundred, Single-leg stretch, Front support (on elbows), Leg pull front (on elbows), Basic back extension, Sphinx, Shoulder bridge prep, Shoulder bridge

REFORMER

Footwork (hold dowel with palms up), Bottom lift, Bottom lift with extension, Arms supine series (in a comfortable range of motion), Hundred prep, Hundred, Coordination, Single-arm coordination, Ab openings, Hip work series, Quadruped abs, Reverse quadruped abs, Scooter, Standing lunge, Seated biceps (arms at comfortable height), Bilateral external rotation, Quadruped triceps kickback, Modified rows, Chest expansion, Shoulder internal rotation, Shoulder external rotation, Prone pulling straps 1, Prone pulling straps 2, Down stretch, Modified balanced control front

CADILLAC

Pelvic curl with RUB, Supine protraction and retraction on foam roll (depending on available range of motion), Assisted squats, Standing arm work series: Chest expansion, Biceps

WUNDA CHAIR

Pelvic curl, Reverse shrugs, Triceps press sit, Prone triceps, Basic swan

	SHOULDER LABRAL TEAR		
Pathology	**General contraindications and precautions**	**Common problems**	**Goals**
Labral tear Shoulder instability	• Use caution with overhead exercises. • Be careful with positions of vulnerability such as combined abduction and external rotation. • Avoid more advanced weight-bearing exercises on long lever (e.g., side bend or up stretch 3 or long stretch).	• Shoulder instability • Shoulder or arm pain with movement and activities • Weak scapular stabilizing muscles • Hypermobile glenohumeral, acromioclavicular, or sternoclavicular joints • History or fear of shoulder subluxating • Limited shoulder function due to apprehension • Clicking or catching sensation with shoulder movement • Poor scapulohumeral rhythm	• Increase strength of scapular stabilizers • Strengthen rotator cuff • Lots of closed-chain exercises, which require cocontraction, thereby promoting joint stability • Restore normal scapulohumeral rhythm • Increase core strength

Recommended exercises

MAT

Pelvic curl, Single-leg lifts, Supine spine twist, Chest lift (variation 4), Chest lift with rotation (variation 4), Hundred prep, Hundred, Single-leg stretch, Front support (on elbows), Leg pull front (on elbows), Side bend (on elbow), Basic back extension, Swimming, Sphinx, Goalpost, Shoulder bridge prep, Shoulder bridge

REFORMER

Footwork (variation 1), Bottom lift, Bottom lift with extension, Arms supine series, Hundred prep, Hundred, Coordination, Single-arm coordination, Ab openings, Quadruped abs, Reverse quadruped abs, Scooter, Seated biceps, Rhomboids 1, Rhomboids 2, Bilateral external rotation, Chest expansion wide, Hug a tree, Quadruped triceps kickback, Modified rows, Chest expansion, Shoulder internal rotation, Shoulder external rotation, Shoulder diagonal pull, Arms overhead, Kneeling biceps, Prone pulling straps 1, Prone pulling straps 2, Up stretch 1, Up stretch 2, Down stretch, Shoulder push, Modified balance control

CADILLAC

Pelvic curl with RUB, Breathing with PTB, Supine protraction and retraction on foam roll, Seated protraction and retraction, Assisted squats, Resisted lunges, Standing arm work series

WUNDA CHAIR

Pelvic curl, Modified swan on floor, Single-arm push-up (quadruped or half plank), Reverse shrugs, Triceps press sit, Prone triceps, Basic swan, Full pike (variation 1)

12

The Hip

The hip is one of the largest joints in the body, has the strongest ligament in the body, and the proximal femur transmits greater loads than any other part of the body. The hip joint structure and its strong but loose fibrous capsule permits it to have the second largest range of movement of all our joints and yet be able to support the weight of the body, arms, and head. As we age, though, hip mobility decreases. Maintenance of adequate hip range of motion is necessary for simple activities of daily living such as walking, running, climbing stairs, sitting, getting up and down from a chair, picking things up off the floor, and tying shoes. Many of the open-chain exercises and stretches in the Pilates repertoire (e.g., hip work series [legs in straps]) address this issue of keeping the hip joints mobile.

Although hip injuries are not as commonly seen as those in the knee or lumbar spine, often dysfunction or weakness of the hips is a contributing or even causative factor for problems in these other areas. For athletes whose activities are primarily in the sagittal plane (running, cycling, flutter kick swimming), I find the Pilates exercises presented in this book especially beneficial, because they challenge the often underused or inhibited frontal plane muscles (glutes and adductors).

The American Association of Hip and Knee Surgeons has stated that with people living longer than ever, arthritis is increasingly more common. It is projected that by 2030, the demand for total hip replacements will grow by 174% to 572,000 in the United States alone. (Kurtz et. al 2007). But most experts agree that low-impact therapeutic exercise (Pilates!) and aquatic exercise are quite effective in reducing pain and prolonging the need for hip replacements.

See the following tables for exercise prescriptions for hip-related conditions. Note that these tables represent what would be generally appropriate for patients with the associated diagnoses or pathologies. However, as every person will present differently and have different issues, it is crucial to assess each client individually and either omit exercises or choose the correct modification as appropriate. If the client does not have the strength, flexibility, or control to perform an exercise correctly, it should not be included in his program.

Exercise Recommendations for Common Hip Injuries and Pathologies

	HIP JOINT REPLACEMENT		
Pathology	General contraindications and precautions	Common problems	Goals
Status post–total hip replacement (hip arthroplasty)	• Specifics vary depending on surgeon and type of hip replacement (approach). Best to consult with surgeon and follow specifics of his or her protocol. • In recent years, many surgeons are using techniques that allow for no weight-bearing precautions and no contraindicated positions. • However, traditionally weight-bearing status and contraindications are non–weight bearing or toe touch weight-bearing for up to six weeks. • For a posterior or posterior lateral approach, avoid hip flexion >90°, hip internal rotation, adduction past a neutral position. • For an anterior approach, avoid a combination of hip extension and external rotation. • All: avoid propulsive and high-impact exercises (no jump board).	• Limited ROM • Stiffness • Muscle tightness • Muscle weakness (primarily abductors and extensors) • Core weakness • Gait abnormalities or antalgic gait • Poor balance or proprioception • Pain	• Restore hip joint ROM • Increase lower extremity (LE) flexibility • Strengthen hip and LE muscles • Improve balance and proprioception • Increase core strength and stability • Normalize gait • Decrease pain and swelling

Recommended exercises

MAT
Pelvic curl, Single-leg lifts, Supine spine twist (variations 1 and 2), Single-leg stretch, Modified single-leg stretch, Front support (variation on elbows), Leg pull front (variation on elbows), Side bend, Swimming, Shoulder bridge prep, Shoulder bridge

REFORMER
Footwork, Bottom lift, Bottom lift with extension, Ab openings, Hip work series, Adductor stretch, Hamstring stretch, Quadruped abs, Scooter, Standing lunge, Up stretch 1, Up stretch 2, Down stretch, Terminal knee extension, Hamstring curl (standing variation only if hip flexion >90° is contraindicated), Skating hybrid, Side splits

CADILLAC
Pelvic curl with RUB, Breathing with PTB, Hip work: double leg supine series, Supine hip flexor stretch with manual assist, Single-leg side series, Assisted squats (with progressions to challenge balance), Resisted lunges, Standing arm work series (with progressions to challenge balance)

WUNDA CHAIR
Pelvic curl, Hamstring curl, Calf press, Standing leg press, Forward lunge (variation 4 to limit the amount of hip flexion; start with variation 1, 2, or 3), Backward step-down (variation 1 or 2), Calf press in forward lunge (variation 1 or 2)

HIP OSTEOARTHRITIS			
Pathology	**General contraindications and precautions**	**Common problems**	**Goals**
Osteoarthritis • Osteoarthrosis • Degenerative joint disease	• Avoid unilateral weight-bearing exercises. • Avoid high-impact exercises. • Avoid heavy loading on the hip joint.	• Pain in the hip, groin, buttock, or thigh • Stiffness • Restricted range of motion (ROM) • Core weakness • Worse upon waking in the morning or after long periods of inactivity • Antalgic gait • Difficulty with ADLs: squatting, dressing, climbing stairs, getting in or out of a car or off or on a chair or toilet • High body weight leads to increased load on the hip joint	• Strengthen hip and lower extremity muscles • Strengthen core muscles • Improve overall flexibility • Decrease load on the hip • Mobilize the hip joint (open-chain exercises)

Recommended exercises

MAT

Pelvic curl, Single-leg lifts, Supine spine twist (variations 1 or 2), Single-leg stretch, Modified single-leg stretch, Front support, Leg pull front, Side bend, Swimming, Shoulder bridge prep, Shoulder bridge

REFORMER

Footwork, Bottom lift, Bottom lift with extension, Ab openings, Hip work series, Adductor stretch, Hamstring stretch, Quadruped abs, Reverse quadruped abs, Up stretch 1 (and elephant variation), Up stretch 2, Down stretch, Shoulder push, Terminal knee extension (seated variation only), Hamstring curl (seated)

CADILLAC

Pelvic curl with RUB, Breathing with PTB, Hip work: double leg supine series, Supine hip flexor stretch with manual assist, Single-leg side series, Assisted squats

WUNDA CHAIR

Pelvic curl, Hamstring curl, Piriformis stretch

HIP BURSITIS			
Pathology	**General contraindications and precautions**	**Common problems**	**Goals**
Bursitis	Avoid positions that put pressure on bursa: • Greater trochanteric—no side lying • Ischiogluteal (IG)—no sitting • Iliopsoas—not too much hip flexor activation	• Pain • Local tenderness over bursa • Limited ROM • Muscle tightness (usually iliotibial band and hip flexor) • LE muscle weakness and imbalances • Core weakness	• Increase LE flexibility • Strengthen weak hip and LE muscles (usually glutes) • Increase core strength and stability • Improve balance and proprioception

Recommended exercises

MAT

Pelvic curl, Single-leg lifts, Supine spine twist, Single-leg stretch, Modified single-leg stretch, Front support, Leg pull front, Side bend, Swimming, Shoulder bridge prep, Shoulder bridge

REFORMER

Footwork, Bottom lift, Bottom lift with extension, Hip work series, Adductor stretch, Hamstring stretch, Quadruped abs, Reverse quadruped abs[a], Scooter, Standing lunge, Quadratus lumborum stretch[b], Up stretch 1, Up stretch 2, Up stretch 3, Long stretch, Down stretch, Terminal knee extension[c], Hamstring curl[d], Skating hybrid, Side splits, Jumping series

CADILLAC

Pelvic curl with RUB, Breathing with PTB, Hip work: double leg supine, Supine hip flexor stretch with manual assist, Single-leg side series, Assisted squats (progression 2, 3, and 4), Resisted lunges, Standing arm work series (with progressions to challenge balance)

WUNDA CHAIR

Pelvic curl, Hamstring curl, Modified swan on floor, Torso press sit[a], Piriformis stretch, Calf press, Standing leg press, Forward lunge, Backward step-down, Calf press in forward lunge, Full pike

[a] Not for iliopsoas

[b] Standing only for ischiogluteal

[c] Standing variation for ischiogluteal, iliopsoas

[d] Not for greater trochanteric

PIRIFORMIS SYNDROME			
Pathology	General contraindications and precautions	Common problems	Goals
Piriformis syndrome	• If symptoms radiate to the foot, follow lumbar disk precautions.	• Pain in hip or buttock area that radiates down the posterior thigh • Local tenderness over piriformis muscle • Weak or inactive gluteal muscles • Overactive, tightened, or shortened hip flexors • Tight hip adductors • Dominant sagittal plane muscles (quads, hamstrings) • Core weakness • Related sacroiliac joint dysfunction • Overpronated feet	• Increase core strength and stability • Strengthen glutes to reduce demand on piriformis • Increase flexibility or length of hip flexors and adductors • Improve hip muscle strength and neuromuscular control • Decrease amount of time spent in seated position

Recommended exercises

MAT

Pelvic curl, Single-leg lifts, Supine spine twist, Chest lift, Chest lift with rotation, Pre-hundred prep, Modified single leg stretch, Front support, Leg pull front, Side bend, Swimming, Shoulder bridge prep, Shoulder bridge

REFORMER

Footwork, Bottom lift (variation 3), Bottom lift with extension (variation 3), Single arm coordination, Hundred prep, Coordination, Ab openings, Hip work series, Adductor stretch, Hamstring stretch, Quadruped abs, Reverse quadruped abs, Scooter, Standing lunge, Quadratus lumborum stretch, Up stretch 1 (and elephant variation), Up stretch 2, Up stretch 3, Long stretch, Down stretch, Skating hybrid, Side splits, Jumping series

CADILLAC

Pelvic curl with RUB (variation 2), Breathing with PTB, Hip work: double leg supine series, Supine hip flexor stretch with manual assist, Single-leg side series, Assisted squats (progression 2, 3, and 4), Resisted lunges, Standing arm work series (with progressions to challenge balance)

WUNDA CHAIR

Pelvic curl (variation 2), Torso press sit, Piriformis stretch, Standing leg press, Forward lunge, Backward step down, Calf press in forward lunge, Full pike

	HIP FLEXOR INJURY		
Pathology	**General contraindications and precautions**	**Common problems**	**Goals**
Hip flexor strain	• Avoid over-working the hip flexors. • Avoid pro-longed sitting.	• Pain in anterior hip area, which may radiate down the front of the thigh • Pain increased with movement—lifting the knee toward the chest • Pain with running, jumping, walking, using stairs • Tight, short hip flexor muscles • Core weakness • Anteriorly tilted pelvis, increased lumbar lordosis	• Strengthen glutes • Increase flexibility or length of hip flexors • Increase core strength and stability • Decrease load on hip flexors by encouraging activation of adductors and pelvic floor muscles • Improve balance and proprioception • Decrease amount of time in sitting position

Recommended exercises

MAT

Pelvic curl (variation 2), Supine spine twist (variations 1 or 2), Chest lift, Chest lift with rotation, Hundred prep, Pre-hundred prep, Modified single-leg stretch, Front support, Leg pull front, Side bend, Swimming, Shoulder bridge prep, Shoulder bridge

REFORMER

Footwork, Bottom lift (variation 3), Bottom lift with extension (variation 3), Coordination, Ab Openings, Hip work series, Adductor stretch, Hamstring stretch, Quadruped abs, Scooter, Standing lunge, Quadratus lumborum stretch, Up stretch 1, Up stretch 2, Up stretch 3, Down stretch, Terminal knee extension, Hamstring curl (standing variation), Skating hybrid, Side splits, Jumping series

CADILLAC

Pelvic curl with RUB (variation 2), Breathing with PTB, Hip work: double leg supine series, Supine hip flexor stretch with manual assist, Single-leg side series, Assisted squats (progression 2, 3, and 4), Resisted lunges, Standing arm work series (with progressions to challenge balance)

WUNDA CHAIR

Pelvic curl (variation 2), Hamstring curl, Piriformis stretch, Calf press, Standing leg press, Forward lunge, Backward step-down, Calf press in forward lunge, Full pike

HIP LABRAL INJURY			
Pathology	**General contraindications and precautions**	**Common problems**	**Goals**

Labral tear or injury
• Can be caused by
  • Trauma
  • Femoro-acetabular impingement
  • Capsular laxity
  • Dysplasia
  • Degeneration
	• Avoid combination of hip flexion and internal rotation.
	• Avoid hip flexor work past 90° of hip flexion.
	• Avoid activities of daily living such as prolonged sitting, running, pivoting on loaded hip, or stair climbing.
	• If the patient is post-operative, follow specific physician protocols, which can vary greatly depending on procedure (arthroscopic excision or debridement or osteotomy).
		• Anterior hip or deep groin pain
		• Hip flexor discomfort
		• Clicking, locking, catching, or giving way
		• Hip joint instability
		• Mild hip ROM limitations (mostly in rotation)
		• Dominant sagittal plane muscles (quads or hamstrings)
		• Excessive hip adduction and internal rotation in functional activities
		• Labral tears are a precursor to early onset osteoarthritis
			• Stabilize hip, pelvis, and core in pain-free positions
			• Optimize alignment of the hip joint and precision of joint motion
			• Restore normal joint ROM
			• Improve hip muscle strength and neuromuscular control
			• Strengthen frontal and transverse plane muscles (hip abductors, deep external rotators, gluteus maximus, and iliopsoas)
			• Improve balance and proprioception
			• Increase core strength and stability
			• Increase LE flexibility to prevent muscle imbalances
			• Decrease amount of time in sitting position

Recommended exercises

MAT

Pelvic curl, Supine spine twist (variations 1 and 2), Chest lift, Chest lift with rotation, Pre-hundred prep, Single-leg stretch, Front support, Leg pull front, Side bend, Swimming, Shoulder bridge prep, Shoulder bridge

REFORMER

Footwork, Bottom lift, Bottom lift with extension, Coordination, Ab openings, Hip work series (smaller ROM), Adductor stretch, Hamstring stretch, Quadruped abs, Reverse quadruped abs, Scooter, Standing lunge, Up stretch 1, Up stretch 2, Up stretch 3, Long stretch, Down stretch, Skating hybrid, Side splits

CADILLAC

Pelvic curl with RUB, Breathing with PTB, Hip work: double leg supine series, Supine hip flexor stretch with manual assist, Single-leg side series, Assisted squats (progression 2, 3, and 4), Resisted lunges, Standing arm work series (with progressions to challenge balance)

WUNDA CHAIR

Pelvic curl, Torso press sit, Standing leg press, Forward lunge, Backward step-down, Calf press in forward lunge, Full pike

13

The Knee

Knee injuries make up the highest percentage of lower extremity injuries, particularly among physically active individuals. The structure of the knee joint makes it inherently unstable, so dynamic stability provided by the muscles and ligaments is crucial. Due to factors such as anatomical differences, less muscular strength and girth, and altered biomechanical patterns, females sustain a higher number of traumatic and overuse knee injuries compared to males.

In recent years it has been well established that proximal factors play a contributory role with respect to knee injuries. A review of biomechanical and clinical studies by biokinesiologist, physical therapist, and leading researcher in this area, Dr. Christopher Powers (2010), indicates that impaired muscular control of the hip, pelvis, and trunk can affect tibiofemoral and patellofemoral joint kinematics in multiple planes. In particular, Powers points to evidence that impairments at the hip may underlie injuries such as anterior cruciate ligament tears, iliotibial band syndrome, and patellofemoral joint pain. Thus, he makes a biomechanical argument for the incorporation of pelvis and trunk stability, as well as dynamic hip joint control, into the design of knee rehabilitation programs. Because all Pilates exercises incorporate pelvic and trunk stability as well as hip control, I find it to be an ideal form of exercise for individuals suffering from knee pathologies.

Postsurgical knee patients often have non–weight-bearing or partial weight-bearing restrictions of up to four weeks. Doing exercises such as footwork on the reformer in the supine position provides zero-gravity spring resistance, thus allowing for progressive load bearing and functional retraining earlier in the rehabilitation period after a surgical procedure. Neuromuscular retraining and functional patterns can be learned for activities such as squatting and lunging in this safe position, so that when the weight-bearing restrictions are lifted, the motions have already been learned. Studies suggest that this may shorten rehabilitation by as much as four weeks, with the largest effect seen within the first two months postoperatively (Mętel, Milert, and Szczygieł 2012).

See the following tables for a summary of exercise prescriptions for patients with knee conditions.

Note that these tables represent what would be generally appropriate for patients with the associated diagnoses or pathologies. However, as every person will present differently and have different issues, it is crucial to assess each client individually and either omit exercises or choose the correct modification as appropriate. If the client does not have the strength, flexibility, or control to perform an exercise correctly, it should not be included in her program.

Exercise Recommendations for Common Knee Injuries and Pathologies

KNEE OSTEOARTHRITIS			
Pathology	**General contraindications and precautions**	**Common problems**	**Goals**
Osteoarthritis • Osteoarthrosis • Degenerative joint disease	• Avoid unilateral weight-bearing exercises. • No heavy load on the knee joint. • Avoid kneeling positions.	• Knee pain • Knee stiffness • Decreased range of motion (ROM) • Swelling • Pain aggravated by weight-bearing activities • Worse pain upon waking in the morning or after long periods of sitting • Weakness of muscles surrounding the knee joint • Antalgic gait • Difficulty with activities of daily living: squatting, dressing, climbing stairs, getting in or out of a car or off or on a chair or toilet • Higher body weight increases load on the knee joint	• Strengthen lower extremity muscles via low load and open-chain exercises • Strengthen core muscles • Improve lower extremity flexibility • Decrease load on knee (lose weight)

Recommended exercises

MAT

Pelvic curl, Single-leg lifts, Single-leg stretch, Modified single leg stretch, Front support (variation on elbows), Leg pull front (variation on elbows), Side bend (variation on elbows), Swimming, Shoulder bridge prep, Shoulder bridge

REFORMER

Footwork (lighter spring, not unilateral if painful), Bottom lift, Bottom lift with extension, Coordination, Single-arm coordination, Ab openings, Hip work series, Adductor stretch, Hamstring stretch, Terminal knee extension (seated variation only), Hamstring curl (seated)

CADILLAC

Pelvic curl with RUB, Breathing with PTB, Hip work: double leg supine series, Supine hip flexor stretch with manual assist, Single-leg side series, Assisted squats

WUNDA CHAIR

Pelvic curl, Hamstring curl, Piriformis stretch

KNEE JOINT REPLACEMENT			
Pathology	**General contraindications and precautions**	**Common problems**	**Goals**
Knee joint replacement • Status post–total knee replacement (knee arthroplasty) • Partial knee joint replacement (unicompartmental)	• Avoid high-impact exercises. • Avoid deep knee bending. • Avoid the kneeling position. • Specifics vary depending on the surgeon and type of knee replacement. It is best to consult with your surgeon and to follow specifics of his or her protocol.	• Limited ROM (especially flexion) • Knee joint stiffness • Knee joint swelling • LE muscle tightness • Muscle weakness (quadriceps, hamstrings, calves, glutes) • Core weakness • Gait abnormalities or antalgic gait • Poor balance and proprioception • Pain	• Restore knee joint ROM • Increase lower extremity (LE) flexibility • Strengthen LE muscles • Improve balance and proprioception • Increase core strength and stability • Normalize gait • Decrease pain and swelling • Retrain functional patterns in partial weight bearing so that when the patient is ready to fully bear weight, the motion has already been learned

Recommended exercises

MAT

Pelvic curl, Single-leg lifts, Single-leg stretch, Modified single-leg stretch, Front support, Leg pull front, Side bend (variation on elbows), Swimming, Shoulder bridge prep, Shoulder bridge

REFORMER

Footwork (with bar high to increase knee flexion), Bottom lift, Bottom lift with extension, Coordination, Single-arm coordination, Ab openings, Hip work series, Adductor stretch, Hamstring stretch, Scooter, Standing lunge (pad under knee), Terminal knee extension, Hamstring curl, Skating hybrid, Side splits

CADILLAC

Pelvic curl with RUB, Breathing with PTB, Hip work: double leg supine series, Supine hip flexor stretch with manual assist, Single-leg side series, Assisted squats (with progressions to challenge balance), Resisted lunges, Standing arm work series (with progressions to challenge balance)

WUNDA CHAIR

Pelvic curl, Hamstring curl, Calf press (with pad under knee), Standing leg press, Forward lunge (variation 4 only to limit the amount of flexion; start with variation 1, 2, or 3), Backward step-down (variation 1 or 2), Calf press in forward lunge (variation 1 or 2)

MENISCAL INJURY			
Pathology	**General contraindications and precautions**	**Common problems**	**Goals**
Meniscus tear • Partial tear • Complete tear • Post–arthroscopic surgery	• Avoid loaded deep knee bending. • Avoid kneeling position. • If the patient is post-op, follow the surgeon's weight-bearing precautions and specific protocol.	• Knee pain • Limited tolerance to sitting • Aggravated by weight-bearing activities (squatting, walking, running), kneeling, and loaded twisting • Locking, popping, clicking • Localized tenderness on the knee • Restricted knee joint ROM • Antalgic gait • Impaired balance and proprioception	• Strengthen all muscles surrounding and supporting the knee joint • Strengthen core muscles • Restore normal ROM • Improve balance and proprioception • Normalize gait

Recommended exercises

MAT

Pelvic curl, Single-leg lift, Single-leg stretch, Modified single leg stretch, Front support, Leg pull front, Side bend, Swimming, Shoulder bridge prep, Shoulder bridge

REFORMER

Footwork (with bar in low position), Bottom lift, Bottom lift with extension, Coordination, Single-arm coordination, Ab openings, Hip work series, Adductor stretch, Hamstring stretch, Scooter, Standing lunge (pad under knee), Up stretch 1, Up stretch 2, Up stretch 3, Long stretch, Terminal knee extension, Hamstring curl, Skating hybrid, Side splits, Standing lunge

CADILLAC

Pelvic curl with RUB, Breathing with PTB, Hip work: double leg supine, Supine hip flexor stretch with manual assist, Single-leg side series, Assisted squats (with progressions to challenge balance), Resisted lunges, Standing arm series (with progressions to challenge balance)

WUNDA CHAIR

Pelvic curl, Hamstring curl, Calf press (pad under patella), Standing leg press, Forward lunge (variation 4 to limit the amount of knee flexion; begin with variation 1, 2, or 3 if needed), Calf press in forward lunge

ANTERIOR CRUCIATE LIGAMENT (ACL) INJURY			
Pathology	**General contraindications and precautions**	**Common problems**	**Goals**
ACL injury • ACL ligament tear (partial or complete) • Status post ACL ligament repair	• No weighted open-chain knee extension. • Avoid twisting maneuvers for the first few months post-op. • Depending on the surgeon and surgical method, there may be weight-bearing precautions as well as specific instructions for return to high-impact activities. Follow the physician's protocol.	• Knee pain • Knee instability • Decreased ROM • Swelling • Weakness of muscles surrounding the knee joint • Lack of eccentric quadriceps strength or control • Poor balance and proprioception • Lengthy rehabilitation and time to return to sport after surgery (six months to one year)	• Decrease swelling • Restore normal knee joint ROM • Strengthen all muscles surrounding and supporting the knee joint • Retrain functional patterns in partial weight bearing so that when the patient is ready to bear weight, the motion has already been learned • Promote knee joint stability (closed-chain exercises) • Strengthen core muscles • Improve balance and proprioception • Increase eccentric quadriceps strength and control

Recommended exercises

MAT

Pelvic curl, Single-leg stretch, Modified single-leg stretch, Front support, Leg pull front, Side bend, Swimming, Shoulder bridge prep, Shoulder bridge

REFORMER

Footwork, Bottom lift, Bottom lift with extension, Coordination, Single-arm coordination, Ab openings, Hip work series, Adductor stretch, Hamstring stretch, Scooter, Standing lunge, Up stretch 1 (elephant variation), Up stretch 2, Terminal knee extension, Hamstring curl, Skating hybrid, Side splits, Jumping series[a]

CADILLAC

Pelvic curl with RUB, Breathing with PTB, Hip work: double leg supine series, Supine hip flexor stretch with manual assist, Single-leg side series, Assisted squats (with progressions to challenge balance), Resisted lunges, Standing arm work series (with progressions to challenge balance)

WUNDA CHAIR

Pelvic curl, Hamstring curl, Calf press, Standing leg press, Forward lunge (begin with variation 1, 2, or 3), Backward step-down (begin with variation 1 or 2), Calf press in forward lunge (begin with variation 1,2 or 3)

[a] Adhere to physician protocol for when the patient can return to high-impact activity.

PATELLOFEMORAL PAIN SYNDROME

Pathology	General contraindications and precautions	Common problems	Goals
Patellofemoral pain syndrome	• Avoid deep knee bends (especially loaded). • Use caution with kneeling and quadruped positions due to pressure on the patella. • Avoid long periods of sitting with knees bent.	• Anterior knee pain • Pain aggravated by sitting with bent knees, squatting, jumping, stairs (especially going down) • Catching, popping, grinding when walking or with open chain movement in and out of flexion • LE muscle imbalance (weak gluteus medius leads to improper patellar tracking) • Tight hamstrings, iliotibial band, or calf muscles • Malalignment or abnormal biomechanics of the hips, knees, or feet • Weakness of muscles surrounding the knee joint • Lack of eccentric quadriceps strength or control	• Strengthen all muscles surrounding and supporting the knee joint • Strengthen frontal plane muscles (primarily gluteus medius) to normalize biomechanics of the hip and pelvis, thereby improving patellar tracking • Strengthen the core muscles • Stretch hamstrings, calves, iliotibial band • Improve balance and proprioception • Increase eccentric quadriceps strength and control

Recommended exercises

MAT

Pelvic curl, Single-leg stretch, Front support, Leg pull front, Side bend, Swimming, Shoulder bridge prep, Shoulder bridge

REFORMER

Footwork, Bottom lift, Bottom lift with extension, Coordination, Ab openings, Hip work series, Adductor stretch, Hamstring stretch, Scooter, Standing lunge (pad under knee), Up stretch 1 (elephant variation), Up stretch 2, Terminal knee extension, Hamstring curl, Skating hybrid, Side splits, Jumping series[b]

CADILLAC

Pelvic curl with RUB, Breathing with PTB, Hip work: double leg supine series, Supine hip flexor stretch with manual assist, Single-leg side series, Assisted squats (with progressions to challenge balance), Resisted lunges, Standing arm work series (with progressions to challenge balance)

WUNDA CHAIR

Pelvic curl, Hamstring curl, Piriformis stretch, Calf press, Standing leg press, Forward lunge (variation 4; begin with variation 1, 2, or 3 if needed), Backward step-down (start with variation 1 or 2), Calf press in forward lunge

[a] When the condition is no longer acute and the patient is returning to her sport.

ILIOTIBIAL BAND SYNDROME			
Pathology	**General contraindications and precautions**	**Common problems**	**Goals**
Iliotibial band syndrome	• Avoid high-impact activities (jumping, running, etc.).	• Lateral knee pain • Pain aggravated by activity (running, jumping) and intensifies over time • Lateral knee instability • LE muscle imbalance (sagittal plane dominant) • Weak hip abductors (primarily gluteus medius) • Overpronated feet • Tight hamstrings, iliotibial band, or calf muscles	• Strengthen frontal plane muscles (primarily gluteus medius) • Strengthen all muscles surrounding and supporting the knee joint • Strengthen core muscles • Stretch hamstrings, calves, quads • Improve balance and proprioception • Promote knee joint stability (closed-chain exercises)

Recommended exercises

MAT

Pelvic curl, Single-leg stretch, Front support, Leg pull front, Side bend, Swimming, Shoulder bridge prep, Shoulder bridge

REFORMER

Footwork, Bottom lift, Bottom lift with extension, Coordination, Ab openings, Hip work series, Adductor stretch, Hamstring stretch, Quadruped abs, Scooter, Standing lunge, Quadratus lumborum stretch, Up stretch 1 (elephant variation), Up stretch 2, Up stretch 3, Terminal knee extension, Hamstring curl, Skating hybrid, Side splits

CADILLAC

Pelvic curl with RUB, Breathing with PTB, Hip work: double leg supine series, Supine hip flexor stretch with manual assist, Single-leg side series, Assisted squats (with progressions to challenge balance), Resisted lunges, Standing arm work series (with progressions to challenge balance)

WUNDA CHAIR

Pelvic curl, Hamstring curl, Piriformis stretch, Calf press, Standing leg press, Forward lunge, Backward step-down, Calf press in forward lunge

PATELLAR TENDINOPATHY			
Pathology	**General contraindications and precautions**	**Common problems**	**Goals**
Patellar tendinopathy • Tendinitis (acute, inflammation) • Tendinosis (chronic, degeneration)	• Avoid high-impact activities (jumping, running, etc.).	• Anterior knee pain (just below the patella) • Pain aggravated by activity (running, jumping • Tightness of the quads or hamstrings • Calf tightness or weakness • Malalignment or abnormal biomechanics of the pelvis or hips • Weak hip abductors (primarily gluteus medius)	• Increase eccentric quadriceps strength and control • Strengthen calf muscles (to help decrease load on patellar tendon when jumping and landing) • Normalize alignment and biomechanics of hip and pelvis (strengthen gluteus medius) • Strengthen core muscles • Stretch hamstrings, quads, and calves • Improve balance and proprioception • Tendinosis: eccentric quadriceps strengthening

Recommended exercises

MAT

Pelvic curl, Hundred prep, Hundred, Single-leg stretch, Front support, Leg pull front, Side bend, Swimming, Shoulder bridge prep, Shoulder bridge

REFORMER

Footwork (in the parallel heels and parallel toes positions, can emphasize eccentric strengthening by pressing out with both legs but returning with only the involved leg)[a], Bottom lift, Bottom lift with extension, Coordination, Ab openings, Hip work series, Adductor stretch, Hamstring stretch, Scooter, Standing lunge (pad under knee), Quadratus lumborum stretch, Up stretch 1 (elephant variation), Up stretch 2, Up stretch 3, Terminal knee extension, Hamstring curl, Skating hybrid, Side splits

CADILLAC

Pelvic curl with RUB, Breathing with PTB, Hip work: double leg supine series, Supine hip flexor stretch with manual assist, Single-leg side series, Assisted squats (with progressions to challenge balance), Resisted lunges, Standing arm work series (with progressions to challenge balance)

WUNDA CHAIR

Pelvic curl, Hamstring curl, Piriformis stretch, Calf press, Standing leg press, Forward lunge[a] (start with variation 1, 2, or 3), Backward step-down (start with variation 1 or 2), Calf press in forward lunge[a] (start with variation)

[a]Not appropriate for acute tendinitis.

14

The Foot and Ankle

Most foot and ankle injuries are from overuse or trauma caused by running, jumping, and cutting in high-impact activities. Therefore, in the early phases of foot and ankle rehab, the Pilates method is an excellent therapeutic exercise to maintain overall strength and general conditioning while the foot and ankle heal. Much of the repertoire can still be done, even with the foot in a cast or boot. In the later stages of foot and ankle rehab, Pilates exercises such as footwork and the jumping series are great tools for relearning proper neuromuscular patterns and functional retraining before returning to one's sport. Physical therapist Deborah Cozen (2001), in her article titled, "Use of Pilates in Foot and Ankle Rehabilitation," states that by incorporating Pilates into the rehabilitation program, a patient's recovery process will be enhanced significantly. She describes Pilates as a functional form of exercise because it combines multiple planes of movement, and she points out that the exercises emphasize muscular balance between opposing muscles and between right and left sides of the body.

Adequate ankle strength and mobility are of course essential for athletes to allow for running, jumping, and cutting, but they are also required for simple daily activities such as walking, balancing on one foot, or getting up and down from a chair. The most important function of the lower leg muscles during gait is the eccentric contractions, or deceleration. For this reason, I find Pilates to be a better method of functional retraining than traditional gym exercises, which tend to emphasize only the concentric phase of the movement. Further, most of our activities of daily living are both open and closed chain. Walking, for example, is closed chain on the stance leg but open chain on the swing leg. Pilates exercises such as scooter (p. 155) and standing leg press (p. 212) simulate this type of action, making it a very functional type of exercise.

With foot and ankle injuries, as with knee injuries, strength and neuromuscular control of the proximal stabilizers (hips, pelvis, and trunk) are very important. We must have adequate stabilization proximally to attain optimal function distally. Unlike traditional physical therapy or gym exercises, Pilates incorporates trunk, pelvic, and hip stability so we are not only strengthening the distal segment (foot) but the entire lower body kinetic chain (figure 14.1).

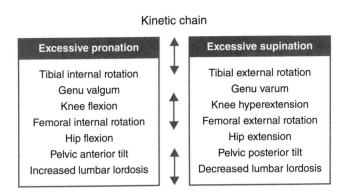

FIGURE 14.1 Lower-body kinetic chain.

See the following tables for a summary of what would be appropriate for patients with foot and ankle conditions.

Note that these tables represent what would be generally be appropriate for patients with these diagnoses or pathologies. However, as every person will present differently and have different issues, it is crucial to assess each client individually and either omit or choose the correct modification as appropriate. If the client does not have the strength, flexibility, or control to perform an exercise correctly, it should not be included in her program.

Exercise Recommendations for Common Ankle and Foot Injuries and Pathologies

ANKLE LIGAMENT INJURY (ANKLE SPRAIN)			
Pathology	**General contraindications and precautions**	**Common problems**	**Goals**

Ankle sprain
• Lateral or inversion sprain (85% of ankle sprains). Can be
  • Mild (grade I)—slight stretch with some fiber damage
  • Moderate (grade II)—Partial tear of ligament
  • Severe (grade III)—complete tear of ligament(s)
• Medial sprain (deltoid ligament). Often accompanied by avulsion fracture and requiring surgery.
• Syndesmotic or high ankle sprain (recovery two to three times longer)
	• Depending on location and grade of sprain, as well as stage of rehab, avoid weight-bearing exercises and excessively supinated or pronated foot positions.	• If acute: pain, swelling, stiffness, throbbing, redness, warmth, other discoloration
		• If chronic: ankle joint laxity or instability
		• Limited ankle ROM
		• Poor balance and proprioception
		• Proximal weakness
		• High rate of recurrence (70%)
			• Decrease swelling and pain
			• Restore normal ankle joint range of motion (ROM)
			• Retrain functional patterns in partial weight bearing so that when the patient is ready to bear weight, the motion has already been learned
			• Promote ankle joint stability (closed-chain exercises)
			• Increase core strength
			• Strengthen proximal muscles
			• Improve balance and proprioception
			• Increase lower leg muscle strength and control

Recommended exercises

MAT

Pelvic curl, Modified single leg (level 2), Front support, Leg pull front, Shoulder bridge prep, Shoulder bridge

REFORMER

Footwork[a], Bottom lift[b], Bottom lift with extension[b], Hip work series, Adductor stretch, Hamstring stretch, Scooter[b], Standing lunge[b], Up stretch 1[b] and elephant variation, Shoulder push[b], Terminal knee extension (acute—seated variation only), Hamstring curl (acute—seated only), Skating hybrid[b], Side splits[b], Jumping series[b] (when returning to sport)

CADILLAC

Pelvic curl with RUB, Hip work: double leg supine series, Supine hip flexor stretch with manual assist, Single-leg side series, Assisted squats (with progressions to challenge balance)[b], Resisted lunges[b], Standing arm work series (with progressions to challenge balance)[b]

WUNDA CHAIR

Pelvic curl, Hamstring curl, Piriformis stretch, Calf press (very light spring for acute stage), Standing leg press[b], Forward lunge[b], Backward step-down[b], Calf press in forward lunge[b], Full pike[b]

[a] Patients in the acute phase can do footwork on the jump board instead of the foot bar.

[b] Not appropriate for acute sprains or postsurgical non- or partial weight bearing patients.

ACHILLES TENDINOPATHY

Pathology	General contraindications and precautions	Common problems	Goals
Achilles tendinopathy • Tendinitis (acute, inflammation) • Tendinosis (chronic, degeneration)	• Avoid running, jumping, and other high-impact exercises.	• Tendinitis: pain, swelling, palpable tenderness, redness, warmth • Tendinosis: chronic pain, localized tendon thickening, irregular structure, and persistent pain with activity • Healing slow due to limited blood supply • Limited ankle ROM • Poor balance and proprioception • Proximal weakness • Shortened or tight calf muscles • Lower leg muscle weakness • Overpronation	• Decrease swelling and pain • Restore normal ankle joint ROM • Gentle stretching of gastrocnemius and soleus • Promote ankle joint stability (closed-chain exercises) • Strengthen proximal muscles • Increase core strength • Improve balance and proprioception • Increase lower leg muscle strength and control • Tendinosis: eccentric calf strengthening

Recommended exercises

MAT

Pelvic curl, Front support, Leg pull front, Shoulder bridge prep, Shoulder bridge

REFORMER

Footwork (in the calf raises position, can emphasize eccentric strengthening by pressing out with both legs but lowering with only the involved leg)[a], Bottom lift, Bottom lift with extension, Hip work series, Adductor stretch, Hamstring stretch, Scooter, Standing lunge, Up stretch 1 and elephant variation, Up stretch 2, Up stretch 3, Long stretch, Down stretch, Shoulder push, Terminal knee extension, Hamstring curl, Skating hybrid, Side splits

CADILLAC

Pelvic curl with RUB, Hip work: double leg supine series, Supine hip flexor stretch with manual assist, Single-leg side series, Assisted squats (with progressions to challenge balance), Resisted lunges, Standing arm work series (with progressions to challenge balance)

WUNDA CHAIR

Pelvic curl, Hamstring curl, Piriformis stretch, Calf press (very light spring for acute stage), Standing leg press, Forward lunge, Backward step-down, Calf press in forward lunge[a], Full pike

[a] Not appropriate for patients with acute tendinitis.

SHIN SPLINTS			
Pathology	**General contraindications and precautions**	**Common problems**	**Goals**
Shin splints • Medial tibial stress syndrome	• Avoid high-impact activities (running, jumping, dancing).	• Pain along the inside lower half of the shin • Pain at the start of high-impact exercise that often eases as the patient continues • Occasionally palpable lumps or swelling • Shortened or tight calf muscles • Relative weakness of anterior lower leg muscle • Overpronation • Proximal weakness (hip external rotators and abductors) • Untreated shin splints can lead to a stress fracture	• Increase anterior lower leg muscle strength and control • Reduce functional overpronation by strengthening the muscles that support the arch of the foot (tibialis posterior and peroneus longus) • Increase core strength • Strengthen proximal muscles (hip external rotators and abductors)

Recommended exercises

MAT

Pelvic curl, Front support, Leg pull front, Shoulder bridge prep, Shoulder bridge

REFORMER

Footwork, Bottom lift, Bottom lift with extension, Hip work series, Adductor stretch, Hamstring stretch, Scooter, Standing lunge, Up stretch 1 (elephant variation), Long stretch, Down stretch, Shoulder push, Terminal knee extension, Hamstring curl, Skating hybrid, Side splits

CADILLAC

Pelvic curl with RUB, Hip work: double leg supine, Supine hip flexor stretch with manual assist, Single-leg side series, Assisted squats (with progressions to challenge balance), Resisted lunges, Standing arm work series (with progressions to challenge balance)

WUNDA CHAIR

Pelvic curl, Hamstring curl, Piriformis stretch, Calf press, Standing leg press, Forward lunge, Backward step-down, Calf press in forward lunge

PLANTAR FASCIITIS			
Pathology	**General contraindications and precautions**	**Common problems**	**Goals**
Plantar fasciitis	• Avoid high-impact activity (running, jumping, dancing)	• Pain along the bottom of the foot or arch • Pain worse first thing in the morning • Aggravated by walking, running, prolonged standing • Irritation and swelling on the plantar surface of the foot • Biomechanical faults such as excessive pronation or heightened arch • Shortened or tight calf muscles	• Reduce functional overpronation by strengthening the muscles that support the arch of the foot (tibialis posterior and peroneus longus) • Strengthen proximal muscles that help prevent overpronation of the foot (hip external rotators and abductors) • Increase core strength • Improve balance and proprioception

Recommended exercises

MAT

Pelvic curl, Front support, Leg pull front, Shoulder bridge prep, Shoulder bridge

REFORMER

Footwork (emphasis on prehensile position), Bottom lift, Bottom lift with extension, Hip work series, Adductor stretch, Hamstring stretch, Scooter, Standing lunge, Arm circles, Kneeling biceps, Up stretch 1 (elephant variation), Up stretch 2, Up stretch 3, Long stretch, Down stretch, Shoulder push, Terminal knee extension, Hamstring curl, Skating hybrid, Side splits

CADILLAC

Pelvic curl with RUB, Hip work: double leg supine, Supine hip flexor stretch with manual assist, Single-leg side series, Assisted squats (with progressions to challenge balance), Resisted lunges, Standing arm work series (with progressions to challenge balance)

WUNDA CHAIR

Pelvic curl, Hamstring curl, Piriformis stretch, Calf press, Standing leg press, Forward lunge, Backward step-down, Calf press in forward lunge, Full pike

REFERENCES

Abe, T., N. Kusuhara, N. Yoshimura, T. Tomita, and P.A. Easton. 1996. Differential respiratory activity of four abdominal muscles in humans. *Journal of Applied Physiology* 80 (April): 1379-89.

Adler, S., D., Beckers, and M. Buck. 1993. *PNF in practice: an illustrated guide*. Berlin Heidelbeg: Spring-Verlag. p. 131.

Akbas, E., and E. U. Erdem. 2016. Does Pilates-based approach provide additional benefit over traditional physiotherapy in the management of rotator cuff tendinopathy? A randomized controlled trial. *Annals of Sports Medicine and Research* 3(6): 1083.

Alfredson, H., and R. Lorentzon. 2000. Chronic Achilles tendinosis: Recommendations for treatment and prevention. *Sports Medicine* 29: 135-46.

Alves de Araujo, M.E., E. Bezerra da Silva, M. Bragade Mello, S.A. Cader, A. Shiguemi Inoue Salgado, and E.H. Dantas. 2012. The effectiveness of the Pilates method: reducing the degree of non-structural scoliosis, and improving flexibility and pain in female college students. *Journal of Bodywork and Movement Therapies* 16(2): 191-8.

Anderson, B., and A. Spector. 2000. Introduction to Pilates-based rehabilitation. *Orthopedic Physical Therapy Clinics of North America* 9 (September): 395-410.

Bahr, R., B. Fossan, S. Loken, and L. J. Engebretsen. 2006. Surgical treatment compared with eccentric training for patellar tendinopathy (jumper's knee): A randomized, controlled trial. *Journal of Bone and Joint Surgery American volume* 88 (8): 1689-98.

Bullock, J., J. Boyle, and M. Wang. 2001. Muscle contraction. In *NMS physiology*, 37-56. 4th ed. Baltimore: Lippincott Williams and Wilkins.

Brourman, S. 2010. Workshop: Using yoga therapeutically. San Pedro, CA.

Cala, S. J., J. Edyvean, and L. A. Engel. 1992. Chest wall and trunk muscle activity during inspiratory loading. *Journal of Applied Physiology* 73 (December): 2373-81.

Campos de Oliveira L, R. Gonçalves de Oliveira, D.A. Pires-Oliveira. 2015. Effects of Pilates on muscle strength, postural balance and quality of life of older adults: a randomized, controlled, clinical trial. *Journal of Physical Therapy Science* 27(3):871–76.

Celik, D., and N. Turkel. 2017. The effectiveness of Pilates for partial anterior cruciate ligament injury. *Knee Surgery, Sports Traumatology, Arthroscopy* 25 (8): 2357-64.

Childs, M.J., J.M. Fritz, S.R. Piva, and J.M. Whitman. 2004. Proposal of a classification system for patients with neck pain. *Journal of Orthopaedic and Sports Physical Therapy* 34 (11): 686-700.

Comerford, M. J., and S. L. Mottram. 2001. Functional stability re-training: Principles and strategies for managing mechanical dysfunction. *Manual Therapy* 6 (1): 3-14.

Cote, P., G. van der Velde, J. D. Cassidy, L. J. Carroll, S. Hogg-Johnson, L. W. Holm, et al. 2008. The burden and determinants of neck pain in workers: Results of the Bone and Joint Decade 2000-2010 Task Force on Neck Pain and its Associated Disorders. *Spine* 33: S60-74.

Cozen, D. M. 2001. Use of Pilates in foot and ankle rehabilitation. *Sports Medicine and Arthroscopy Review* 8 (October-December): 395-403.

De Troyer, A., M. Estenne, V. Ninane, D. Van Gansbeke, and M. Gorini. 1990. Transversus abdominis muscle function in humans. *Journal of Applied Physiology* 68 (March): 1010-16.

Donatelli, R. 2009. Golf: Conditioning for the hip/trunk and compensatory swing mechanics. Educata online seminars. http://www.educata.com/professorprofile.aspx?i=11

Dunleavey, K., K. Kava, A. Goldberg, M. H. Malek, S. A. Talley, V. Tutag-Lehr, and J. Hildreth. 2016. Comparative effectiveness of Pilates and yoga group exercise interventions for chronic mechanical neck pain: Quasi-randomised parallel controlled study. *Physiotherapy* 102: 236-42.

Ekstrom, R. A., R. A. Donatelli, and K. C. Carp. 2007. Electromyographic analysis of core trunk, hip, and thigh muscles during 9 rehabilitation exercises. *Journal of Orthopaedic and Sports Physical Therapy* 37 (12): 754-61.

Emery, K., S. J. De Serres, A. McMillan, and J. N. Cote. 2010. The effects of a Pilates training program on arm-trunk posture and movement. *Clinical Biomechanics* 25: 124-30.

Endleman, I., and D. J. Critchley. 2008. Transversus abdominis and obliquus internus activity during Pilates exercises: Measurement with ultrasound scanning. *Archives of Physical Medicine and Rehabilitation* 89: 2205-12.

Ferreira, P.H, M.L. Ferreira, C.G. Maher, R.D. Herbert, and K. Refshauge. 2006. Specific stabilization exercise for spinal and pelvic pain: a systematic review. Australian Journal of Physiotherapy 52(2): 79-88.

Geriland, J. 1996. Go with the flow (Mihaly Csikzentmihaly interview). *Wired.* September 1, 196. https://www.wired.com/1996109/czik/. Accessed March 19, 2018.

Herrington, L., and R. Davies. 2005. The influence of Pilates training on the ability to contract the transversus abdominis muscle in asymptomatic individuals. *Journal of Bodywork and Movement Therapies* 9 (1): 52-57.

Hides, J. A., C. A. Richardson, and G. A. Jull. 1996. Multifidus muscle recovery is not automatic after resolution of acute, first-episode low back pain. *Spine* 21 (23): 2763-69.

Hides, J., W. Stanton, M. D. Mendis, and M. Sexton. 2011. The relationship of transversus abdominis and lumbar multifidus clinical muscle tests in patients with chronic low back pain. *Manual Therapy* 16 (6): 573-77.

Hodges, P. W., and S. C. Gandevia. 2000. Changes in intra-abdominal pressure during postural and respiratory activation of the human diaphragm. *Journal of Applied Physiology* 89 (September): 967-76.

Hodges, P. W., and C. A. Richardson. 1996. Inefficient muscular stabilization of the lumbar spine associated with low back pain. A motor control evaluation of transversus abdominis. *Spine* 21 (November): 2640-50.

Hodges, P. W., and C. A. Richardson. 1998. Delayed postural contraction of transversus abdominis in low back pain associated with movement of the lower limb. *Journal of Spinal Disorders* 11 (February): 46-56.

Hodges, P. W., and C. A. Richardson. 1999. Transversus abdominis and the superficial abdominal muscles are controlled independently in a postural task. *Neuroscience Letters* 265 (2): 91-94.

Hoy, D., L. March, A. Woolf, F. Blyth, P. Brooks, E. Smith, et al. 2014. The global burden of neck pain: Estimates from the global burden of disease 2010 study. *Annals of the Rheumatic Diseases* 73: 1309-15.

Isacowitz, R. 2005. *Body Arts and Science International movement analysis workbooks (reformer, wunda chair and ladder barrel, Cadillac, auxiliary, mat).* Costa Mesa, CA: Body Arts and Science International.

Isacowitz, R. 2006. *Achieving core strength at every level of the Pilates repertoire. Workshop handout.* Ventura, CA.

Isacowitz, R. 2006. *Pilates, biomechanics and reality. Positive biomechanical concepts can transform into negative movement patterns. Workshop handout.* Costa Mesa, CA.

Isacowitz, R. 2008. *Comprehensive course study guide.* Costa Mesa, CA: Body Arts and Science International.

Isacowitz, R. 2013. *Powerhouse of the upper girdle. Workshop handout.* Costa Mesa, CA.

Isacowitz, R. 2014. *Pilates.* 2nd ed. Champaign, IL: Human Kinetics.

Isacowitz, R. 2018. *Body Arts and Science International movement analysis workbooks (reformer, wunda chair and ladder barrel, Cadillac, auxiliary, mat).* Costa Mesa, CA: Body Arts and Science International.

Isacowitz, R. 2018. *The Mentor Program course manual.* Costa Mesa, CA: Body Arts and Science International.

Isacowitz, R. 2018. *Master I Program course manual.* Costa Mesa, CA: Body Arts and Science International.

Isacowitz, R. 2018. *Master II Program course manual.* Costa Mesa, CA: Body Arts and Science International.

Isacowitz, R., and K. Clippinger. 2011. *Pilates anatomy.* Champaign, IL: Human Kinetics.

Jull, G. A., S. P. O'Leary, and D. L. Falla. 2008. Clinical assessment of the deep cervical flexor muscles: The craniocervical flexion test. *Journal of Manipulative Physiological Therapeutics* 31 (7): 525-33.

Jull, G. A., and C. A. Richardson. 2000. Motor control problems in patients with spinal pain: A new direction for therapeutic exercise. *Journal of Manipulative Physiological Therapy* 23(February): 115-17.

Jull, G. A., P. Trott, H. Potter, G. Zito, K. Niere, D. Shirley, J. Emberson, I. Marschner, and C. Richardson. 2002. A randomized controlled trial of exercise and manipulative therapy for cervicogenic headache. *Spine* 27: 1835-43.

Kamkar, A., J.J. Irrgang, and S.L. Whitney. 1993. Nonoperative management of secondary shoulder impingement syndrome. *Journal of Orthopaedic and Sports Physical Therapy* 17(5):212-24.

Kao, Y. H., T. H. Liou, Y. C. Huang, Y. W. Tsai, and K. M. Wang. 2015. Effects of a 12-week Pilates course on lower limb muscle strength and trunk flexibility in women living in the community. *Health Care for Women International* 36 (3): 303-19.

Klein, G. R., B. R. Levine, W. J. Hozack, E. J. Strausse, J. A. D'Antonio, W. Macaulay, and P. E. Di Cesare. 2007. Return to athletic activity after total hip arthroplasty. Consensus guidelines based on a survey of the Hip Society and American Association of Hip and Knee Surgeons. *Journal of Arthroplasty* 22: 171-75.

Kloubec, J. A. 2010. Pilates for improvement of muscle endurance, flexibility, balance and posture. *Journal of Strength and Conditioning Research* 24 (March): 661-67.

Kolar, P., J. Sulc, M. Kyncl, J. Sanda, O. Cakrt, R. Andel, K. Kumagai, and A. Kobesova. 2012. Postural function of the diaphragm in persons with and without chronic low back pain. *Journal of Orthopaedic and Sports Physical Therapy* 42 (4): 352-62.

Kuo, Y. L., E. A. Tully, and M. P. Galea. 2009. Sagittal spinal posture after Pilates-based exercise in healthy older adults. *Spine* 34 (May): 1046-51.

Kurtz S., K. Ong, E. Lau, F. Mowat, and M. Halpern. 2007. Projections of primary and revision hip and knee arthroplasty in the United States from 2005 to 2030. *Journal of Bone and Joint Surgery. American Volume* 89(4): 780-5.

Lee S., C. Lee, D. O'Sullivan, J. Jung, and J. Park. 2016. Clinical effectiveness of a Pilates treatment for forward head posture. *Journal of Physical Therapy Science* 28 (7): 2009-13.

Levine, B., B. Kaplanek, and W. L. Jaffe. 2009. Pilates training for use in rehabilitation after total hip and knee arthroplasty: A preliminary report. *Clinical Orthopaedics and Related Research* 467: 1468-75.

Limba da Fonseca, J., M. Magini, and T. de Freitas. 2009. Laboratory gait analysis in patients with low back pain before and after a Pilates intervention. *Journal of Sport Rehabilitation* 18: 269-82.

Lugo-Larcheveque, N., L. S. Pescatello, T. W. Dugdale, D. M. Veltri, and W. O. Roberts. 2006. Management of lower extremity malalignment during running with neuromuscular retraining of the proximal stabilizers. *Current Sports Medicine Reports* 5 (May): 137-40.

Lumley, M. A., J. L. Cohen, G. S. Borszcz, A. Cano, A. M. Radcliffe, L. S. Porter, et al. 2011. Pain and emotion: A biopsychosocial review of recent research. *Journal of Clinical Psychology* 67: 942-68.

Machado G.C., C.G. Maher, P.H. Ferreira, J. Latimer, B.W. Koes, D. Steffens, and M.L. Ferreira. 2017. Can recurrence after an acute episode of low back pain be predicted? *Physical Therapy*. 97 (9): 889-895.

Mafi, N., R. Lorentzon, and H. Alfredson. 2001. Superior short-term results with eccentric calf muscle training compared to concentric training in a randomized prospective multicenter study on patients with chronic Achilles tendinosis. *Knee Surgery, Sports Traumatology, Arthroscopy* 9: 42-47.

Metel, S., A. Milert, and E. Szczygieł. 2012. Pilates based exercise in muscle disbalances prevention and treatment of sports injuries: An international perspective on topics in sports medicine and sports injury. K. R. Zaslav (Ed.). *InTech*, doi:10.5772/25557.

Moffett J. and S. McLean. 2006. The role of physiotherapy in the management of non-specific back pain and neck pain. *Rheumatology* 45: 371-78.

Natour, J., L. Araujo Cazotti, L.H. Ribeiro, A. S. Baptista, and A. Jones. 2015. Pilates improves pain, function and quality of life in patients with chronic low back pain: A randomized controlled trial. *Clinical Rehabilitation* 29 (1): 59-68.

Oliveira, L. C., C.A. Guedes, F.J. Jassi, F.A.N. Martini, and R.G. Oliveira. 2016. Effects of the Pilates method on variables related to functionality of a patient with a traumatic spondylolisthesis at L4-L5: A case study. *Journal of Bodywork and Movement Therapies* 20 (January): 123-31.

Orozco-Levi, M., J. Gea, J. Monells, X. Aran, M.C. Aguar, and J.M. Broquetas. 1995. Activity of latissimus dorsi muscle during inspiratory threshold loads. *European Respiratory Journal* 8: 441-45.

Page, P., C. Frank, and R. Lardner. 2010. *Assessment and treatment of muscle imbalance: the Janda approach.* Champaign, IL: Human Kinetics.

Page, P. 2011. Cervicogenic headaches: An evidence-led approach to clinical management. *International Journal of Sports Physical Therapy* 6 (3): 254-66.

Paine, R., and M. L. Voight. 2013. The role of the scapula. *International Journal of Sports Physical Therapy* 8 (5): 617-29.

Pilates, J. H. 1945. *Return to life through contrology.* Miami, FL: Pilates Method Alliance.

Powers, C. 2010. The influence of abnormal hip mechanics on knee injury: A biomechanical perspective. *Journal of Orthopaedic and Sports Physical Therapy* 40 (February): 42-51.

Richardson, C. A., C.J. Snijders, J.A. Hides, L. Damen, M.S. Pas, and J. Storm. 2002. The relation between the transversus abdominis muscles, sacroiliac joint mechanics and low back pain. *Spine* 27 (4): 339-405.

Richardson, C., G. Jull, and P. Hodges. 2004. *Therapeutic exercise for spinal segmental stabilization.* 2nd ed. London: Churchill Livingstone.

Rydeard, R., A. Leger, and D. Smith. 2006. Pilates-based therapeutic exercise: Effect on subjects with nonspecific chronic low back pain and functional disability; A randomized controlled trial. *Journal of Orthopaedic and Sports Physical Therapy* 36 (July): 472-84.

Sapsford, R.R., P.W.Hodges, C.A. Richardson, D.H. Cooper, S.J. Markwell, and G.A. Hull. 2001. Co-activation of the abdominal and pelvic floor muscles during voluntary exercises. *Neurourology and Urodynamics* 20 (1): 31-42.

Seeto, W. 2011. Pilates for injury recovery. *Advance for Physical Therapy and Rehab Medicine.* http://physical-therapy.advanceweb.com/Features/Articles/Pilates-for-Injury-Recovery.aspx (Last updated July 15, 2011).

Segal, N. A., J. Hein, and J. R. Basford. 2004. The effects of Pilates training on flexibility and body composition: An observational study. *Archives of Physical Medicine and Rehabilitation* 85 (December): 1977-80.

Sekendiz, B., O. Altun, F. Korkusuz, and S. Akin. 2007. Effects of Pilates exercise on trunk strength, endurance and flexibility in sedentary adult females. *Journal of Bodywork and Movement Therapies* 11 (October): 318-26.

Troup J.D., J.W. Martin, and D.C. Lloyd. 1981. Back pain in industry. A prospective survey. *Spine* 6 (1): 61-9.

Tsao, H., and P. W. Hodges. 2007. Immediate changes in feedforward postural adjustments following voluntary motor training. *Experimental Brain Research* 181 (4): 537-46.

Urquhart, D. M., P. W. Hodges, T. J. Allen, and I. H. Story. 2005. Abdominal muscle recruitment during a range of voluntary exercises. *Manual Therapy* 10: 144-53.

Viera, F. T., L. M. Faria, J. I. Wittmann, W. Teixeira, and L. A. Nogueira. 2013. The influence of Pilates method in quality of life of practitioners. *Journal of Bodywork Movement Therapies* 17: 483-87.

Wells, C., G. Kolt, P. Marshall, B. Hill, and A. Bialocerkowski. 2014. The effectiveness of Pilates exercise in people with chronic low back pain: A systematic review. *PLoS ONE* 9 (7): e100402. doi:10.1371/journal.pone.0100402.

Wilson, J.D., C.P. Dougherty, M.L. Ireland, and I.M. Davis. 2005. Core stability and its relationship to lower extremity function and injury. *Journal of the American Academy of Orthopaedic Surgeons* 13(5):316-25.

Withers, G. and B. Bryant. 2011. *Introducing APPI Pilates for rehabilitation: Matwork level 1 course workbook.* Fresno, CA.

Wood, S. 2004. A cash-based Pilates niche can boost your bottom line. Advance for Physical Therapists. 15(10) (April 26, 2004): 49.

Zazulak, B.T, T. E. Hewett, N. P. Reeves, B. Goldberg, and J. Cholewicki. 2007. Deficits in neuromuscular control of the trunk predict knee injury risk: A prospective biomechanical-epidemiologic study. *American Journal of Sports Medicine* 35 (7): 1123-30.

INDEX

Note: The italicized *f* and *t* following page numbers refer to figures and tables, respectively.

ABOUT THE AUTHOR

Samantha Wood, MPT, MBA, PMA-CPT, RYT, is a licensed physical therapist, a Pilates Method Alliance–certified Pilates instructor, a Yoga Alliance–certified teacher, and an associate faculty member for BASI Pilates. She has been a member of the American Physical Therapy Association (APTA) since 1997 and of the Pilates Method Alliance (PMA) and Yoga Alliance since 2010. She is the owner of The Cypress Center in Pacific Palisades, California, where she and her staff integrate Pilates with physical therapy for people of all ages and abilities. Her clinical expertise includes Pilates-based rehabilitation, yoga therapy, orthopedics, sports therapy, and functional rehabilitation.

Courtesy of Kelly M. Thomas Photography.

Wood received her bachelor's degree in exercise science from USC in 1991, where she worked as a student athletic trainer with athletes from all sports, specializing in volleyball, football, and track. After graduation she worked as a fitness instructor for Golden Door Spa aboard Cunard cruise ships. Two years later she earned a master of physical therapy (MPT) degree from Western University of Health Sciences. She also holds an MBA from the University of Southern California (USC). She has worked with many celebrities and professional athletes. While at HealthSouth in Arizona, she was the physical therapist for the Phoenix Suns, Phoenix Coyotes, Phoenix Mercury, and Arizona Rattlers. In 2010, she was selected as the physical therapist for the EAS Unstoppable Tour, where her responsibilities included keeping elite athlete Sam Tickle in top physical condition as he completed his 30-sport, 30-city, 30-day journey.

Wood began her Pilates studies in 2001 with Rael Isacowitz and has attended many of Isacowitz's advanced courses, including the prestigious mentor and master programs. She created and teaches two advanced education courses for BASI Pilates: Pilates for Injuries and Pathologies (for Pilates teachers) and Pilates: Integration Into Therapeutic Practice (for rehabilitation professionals). She has been presenting those courses, in addition to offering other workshops and lectures at Pilates conferences around the world, since 2010.

Wood has been featured in the "Ask the Expert" column in *Pilates Style* magazine and authored and modeled for an article entitled "Check In to (Injury) Rehab." She also wrote an article about integration of Pilates into a physical therapy practice for *Advance for Physical Therapists*.

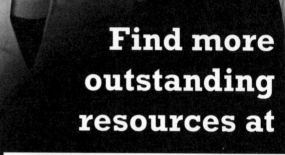

Find more outstanding resources at

www.HumanKinetics.com

In the **U.S.** call 1-800-747-4457
Canada 1-800-465-7301
U.K./Europe +44 (0) 113 255 5665
International 1-217-351-5076

eBook
available at
HumanKinetics.com

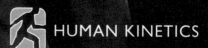

HUMAN KINETICS